Medicine and Public Health through Time

For AQA GCSE Specification A

Derek Patterson
Editor: J.A. Cloake

Hodder Murray

A MEMBER OF THE HODDER HEADLINE GROUP

The publishers would like to thank the following individuals, institutions and companies for permission to reproduce copyright illustrations in this book:

Mary Evans Picture Library: p3; Museum and Arts service of the Doncaster Metropolitan Borough Council Education Services: p4; Hulton Getty: p5, p46 (right), p49; AKG London: p9 (top), p19 (top, left), p20; Collection of Musée de l'Homme: p9 (bottom); E D Hoppé/ Corbis: p10; Chris Hellier/CORBIS: p11; Photo RMN-Hervé Lewandowski, Louvre: p.13; Araldo de Luca/CORBIS: p.14; English Heritage Photo Library/ Jeremy Edwards: p.16; English Heritage Photo Library/Jonathan Bailey: p17; AKG London/Erich Lessing (Paris, Musée du Louvre): p18 (left and right); Wellcome Library, London: p19 (top and bottom, right), p29 (top), p37 (top and bottom), p52; Foto Roncaglia: p28 (left); Bodleian Library: p28 (right): Österreichische Nationalbibliothek: p29 (bottom); Sonia Halliday Photographs: p32; Masters and Fellows of Trinity College, Cambridge: p33; Bettman/Corbis: p38; British Library: p40 (top and bottom); Hulton Archive: p45 (top); Science Museum/Science & Society Picture Library: p45 (bottom); The Bond McIndoe Centre, Queen Victoria Hospital: p46 (left); National Medical Slide Bank/Wellcome: p54 (top); Corbis: p54 (bottom); Alfred Pasieka/Science Photo Library: p55; Frognal Centre, Queen Mary's Hospital, Sidcup, Kent: p56; Sir William Dunn School of Pathology, University of Oxford: p57; PA Photos: p58.

Every effort has been made to trace and acknowledge ownership of copyright. The publishers will be glad to make suitable arrangements with any copyright holders whom it has not been possible to contact.

Note about the Internet links in the book. The user should be aware that URLs or web addresses change regularly. Every effort has been made to ensure the accuracy of the URLs provided in this book on going to press. It is inevitable, however, that some will change. It is sometimes possible to find a relocated web page, by just typing in the address of the home page for a website in the URL window of your browser.

Orders: please contact Bookpoint Ltd, 130 Milton Park, Abingdon, Oxon OX14 4SB. Telephone: (44) 01235 827720. Fax: (44) 01235 400454. Lines are open from 9.00 - 5.00, Monday to Saturday, with a 24 hour message answering service. You can also order through our website www.hoddereducation.co.uk

British Library Cataloguing in Publication Data
A catalogue record for this title is available from the British Library

ISBN (10) 0 340 846 399
ISBN (13) 978 0 340 84639 1

First Published 2003
Impression number   10 9 8 7 6 5 4 3
Year   2009 2008 2007
Copyright © 2003 Derek Patterson, J.A. Cloake

The cover photo shows 'The Stone of Madness' by Brueghel, The Bridgman Art Library.
Typeset by Pantek Arts Ltd, Maidstone, Kent.
Printed for Hodder Murray, an imprint of Hodder Education, a member of the Hodder Headline group, 338 Euston Road, London NW1 3BH by Hobbs the Printer, Totton, Hants.

A Student Guide to Examination and Assessment (AQA Specification History A GCSE)

The examination is a test of your ability to explain what you have understood and to show what you have learnt from studying *Medicine and Public Health through Time*. This may seem obvious. What is not so obvious is how the understanding and knowledge that you show in your examination answer booklet is assessed and marked.

Examiners carry out the assessment and marking of your answers. They are instructed to give marks for specific things that you have written. The purpose of this book is to help you to understand what the examiner is looking for so that you can improve your final grade.

Examiners look for answers which:

- are well explained and clearly organised with good spelling and punctuation (all questions);
- use accurate and relevant knowledge to show what you have learnt (most questions);
- understand what a source does or does not show about developments in medicine (particular questions in Sections A, B and C);
- discuss the good and bad points about an interpretation of an event in the development of medicine (particular questions in Section A).

The examination paper will be divided into three sections.

SECTION A – Medicine through Time (specified topic)

Compulsory source-based question with four or five parts based on four or five sources. It will test your knowledge and understanding of a specific topic. Your school is told which topic before you begin your course.

▶ **SOURCE A**

Cartoon against smallpox vaccinations

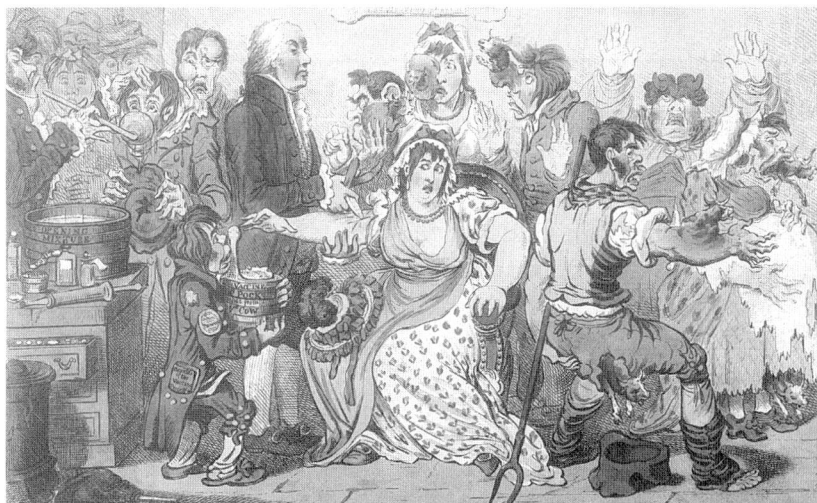

- For 2003: 'Developments in the prevention of disease in the eighteenth and nineteenth centuries'.
- For 2004: 'The impact of religion on medicine in the Middle Ages'.
- For 2005: 'The impact of science and technology on medicine since 1900'.

Here is an example of a question that might be used as the first part of Section A.

Consider this question

How does Source A help you to understand why people opposed smallpox vaccination?
(5 marks)

Comments

The question is asking you to show an understanding of what the source is about by using comprehension and inference based on the source. To reach the top level you would need to make an *inference*, which means you have to explain how you have reached your opinion by reasoning or making a conclusion from the source alone.

SECTION B – Medicine through Time (10 000 BC to the present day)

Compulsory question with a **choice of one from two**. Each choice will have two parts. One will be based on a source. The other will ask for knowledge of the changes in:

- cause and cure;
- anatomy and surgery.

Here is an example of a question that might be used as the second part of a question in Section B.

Consider this question

How important was the work of Hippocrates in explaining the cause and cure of disease at the time of the Ancient Greeks and Romans?

Support your answer with reasons and examples. **(12 marks)**

Comments

This is a question about the role of an individual as a factor in the development of medicine in ancient times. A good answer would show knowledge of the work of Hippocrates. Better answers would also show knowledge of other factors that encouraged change in medical ideas at the time.

These other factors might be:

- the ideas of other Greek thinkers;
- the failure of supernatural ideas to explain and cure disease.

The best answers would explain why one factor was more important than another in a short conclusion.

SECTION C – Public Health in Britain (from the Roman period to the present day)

Compulsory question with a **choice of one from two**. Each choice will have three parts. One of the parts will be based on a source.

Here is an example of a question that might be used as the source-based part of a question in Section C.

▶ SOURCE A

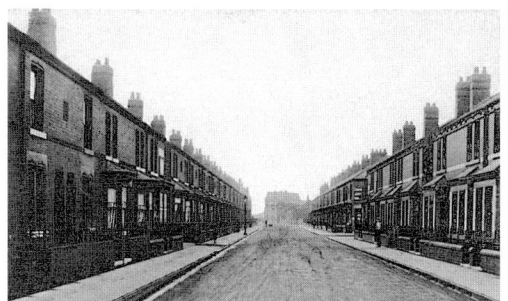

Terraced housing in Doncaster

Consider this question

What can you learn from Sources A and B about improvements in public health during the early twentieth century?

Explain your answer using the sources and your own knowledge.
(5 marks)

Comments

This question asks you to use the sources and your knowledge. You need to use both in order to produce a good answer. The sources show some development but from your own knowledge you should also know that the First World War happened during this period and that it led to some changes.

▲ SOURCE B

Council housing in Essex

How will my answers be assessed and marked?

General points about what the examiner is looking for can be found on page 3.

What examiners do:

- They use a mark scheme drawn up by the people who set the examination paper.
- They check your answers against this mark scheme.
- They award a level for things you have written that fit the mark scheme.
- They decide how many marks to give your answer within the level you have reached.
- They write the marks and the level on your answer.
- They do not take marks off for things you have got wrong.

This is an example of a mark scheme that goes with the question on Section A on pages 5–6.

Consider this question again

How does Source A help you to understand why people opposed smallpox vaccination? (5 marks)

Target: Comprehension and inference (opinion that is explained) from an historical source

Level 1: Answer that selects detail from the source (1 mark)
E.g. The cartoon shows cows growing out of peoples' bodies.

Level 2: Answer that draws a simple inference from the source (2–3 marks)

E.g. There are cows growing out of peoples' bodies and this shows that they were frightened of the side effects of vaccination.

Level 3: Answer that develops a complex inference from the source (4–5 marks)

E.g. This is a cartoon and it is clearly making fun of vaccination by showing cows growing out of peoples' bodies. It may be that some people were frightened of the side-effects of the vaccine but as this is only one source it is hard to get a general picture of why people generally opposed vaccination.

Comments

Examiners have to decide which level your answer is in. If they put your answer in Level 2 or Level 3 they then have to decide how many marks to give it. This will depend on several things such as:

- how well it is written and explained;
- how many convincing reasons you have given;
- how many accurate and relevant facts you have used to support your answer.

How many marks would you give the example answer for Level 3?

What questions will be asked?

Only the people who set the examination paper know the exact questions but they are not trying to trick you. They can only set questions on:

- the content of the course;
- the three assessment objectives.

You can revise the content of the course by using a textbook or working on your class and homework notes.

The assessment objectives shape this content into questions. These questions are fairly predictable.

Assessment Objective 1 – Deployment of knowledge

This simply means that you are expected to have remembered what you have learnt and to have used it in the right place on the examination paper. The kinds of questions you might be asked are:

- What caused something to change in medicine at a particular time?

- What were the results of an event or action in the history of medicine?
- What factors contributed to change? (War, superstition, religion, chance, government, science and technology, the work of individuals.)
- How quickly or slowly did medicine change at different times? (Progress, regress, continuity.)

Assessment Objective 2 – Use of sources

You need to use the sources in your answers when you are asked to do so. Do not rely totally on a source. Always compare a source with what you know or with another source or both depending on the wording of the question.

The kinds of things you might be asked are:

- How does Source Y help you to understand medicine at the time?

- How does Source X show that ideas about medicine had changed?
- What does Source Z tell you about medicine?
- What can you learn from Source T about medicine?

Look at the mark scheme on pages 5–6 and think about how you might write a good answer to these questions. Invent some questions of your own and try them on your friends.

Assessment Objective 3 – Interpretations and representations of the past

Questions testing this objective are usually the most difficult to answer:

- They will involve looking at at least two sides or views about a development in medicine.
- You will have to consider both views by showing you understand and have knowledge of them.
- The answer will involve extended writing.
- You will need to finish by deciding which side the evidence you have presented supports.
- Answers will often involve the use of sources as well as your own knowledge.

The kind of questions you might be asked are:

'Religion hindered the development of medicine in the middle ages'. Explain why you agree or disagree with this interpretation.

'Developments in surgery after 1900 were mainly the result of scientific discoveries made between 1850 and 1895'. Do you agree? Use the sources and your knowledge to help you to explain your answer.

Some questions will involve all objectives.

Revision Tips

What you write and the way you write it is very important. If examiners cannot understand what you are trying to say then they cannot award marks for your answer. **Learn to use and spell key words correctly.**

1. Medicine in the Ancient World

A summary of what you need to know about the ancient world

Exam Paper		Sections A and B	Sections A and B	Section C
Time	Theme	Cause, prevention and cure of disease and infection	Practices of anatomy and surgery	Public health in Britain
10 000 BC		Prehistoric societies and beliefs Ancient Egypt	Trephinning Mummification Attitudes to human dissection	
Ancient world		Ancient Greece • Aristotle • Asklepios • Hippocrates • Alexandria Ancient Rome • Greek influence • Public health • Galen		Facilities in the Roman period
AD 500		• Impact of the fall of Rome	The works of Galen	

✏️ Revision Tips

Time charts such as the one above are helpful because they give you a quick and easy way of checking what you need to know.

You need to make your own revision time charts, which give a little more detail about each of the people or events shown. When you have reduced your charts to the details shown on the one above you will be ready to do well in the examination. **Do it now.**

The first area you need to study is the key features of prehistoric society. The reason you need to know something about this is so that you can show an understanding of how medicine developed during the time of:

• Ancient Egypt
• Ancient Greece
• Ancient Rome.

Look carefully at the three picture sources on the next two pages.

Key features of prehistoric society

Prehistoric surgery

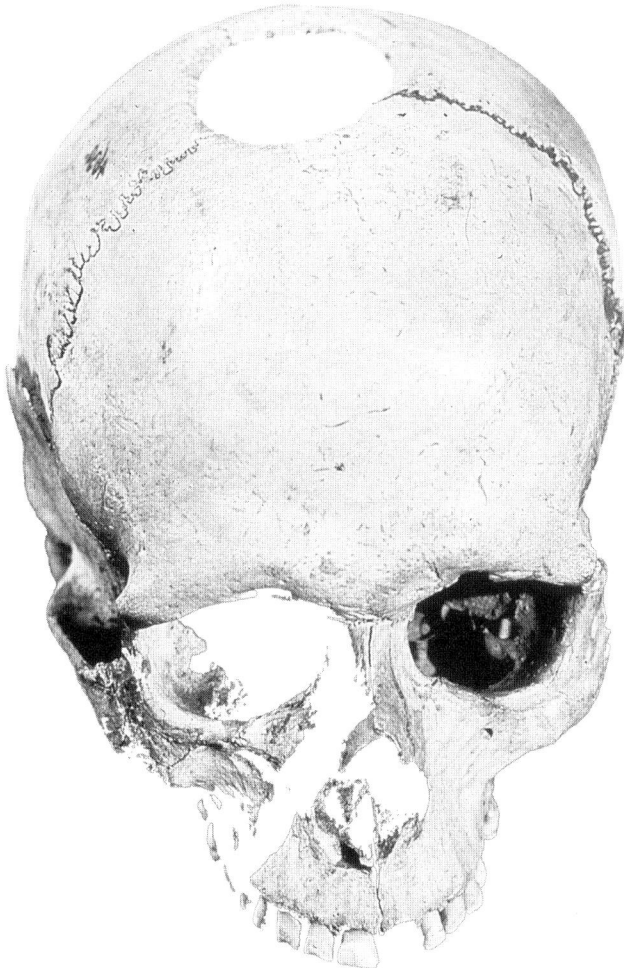

◄ **SOURCE A**

Picture of a trephined skull

Prehistoric magic and superstition

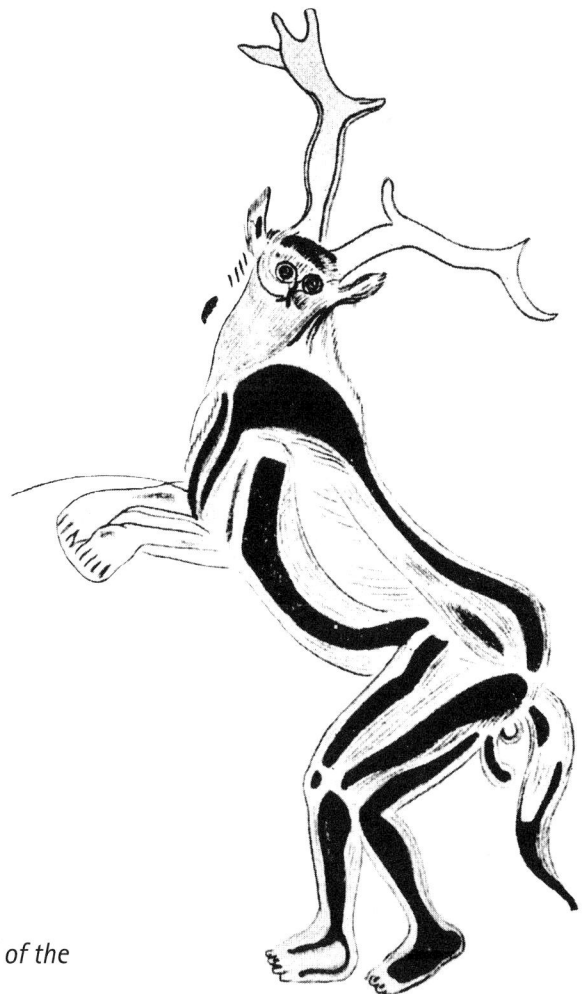

▶ **SOURCE B**

Picture of the strange figure painted on the wall of the Three Brothers Cave in France

Prehistoric lifestyles

▼ SOURCE C

Picture of an Australian Aborigine living in modern times

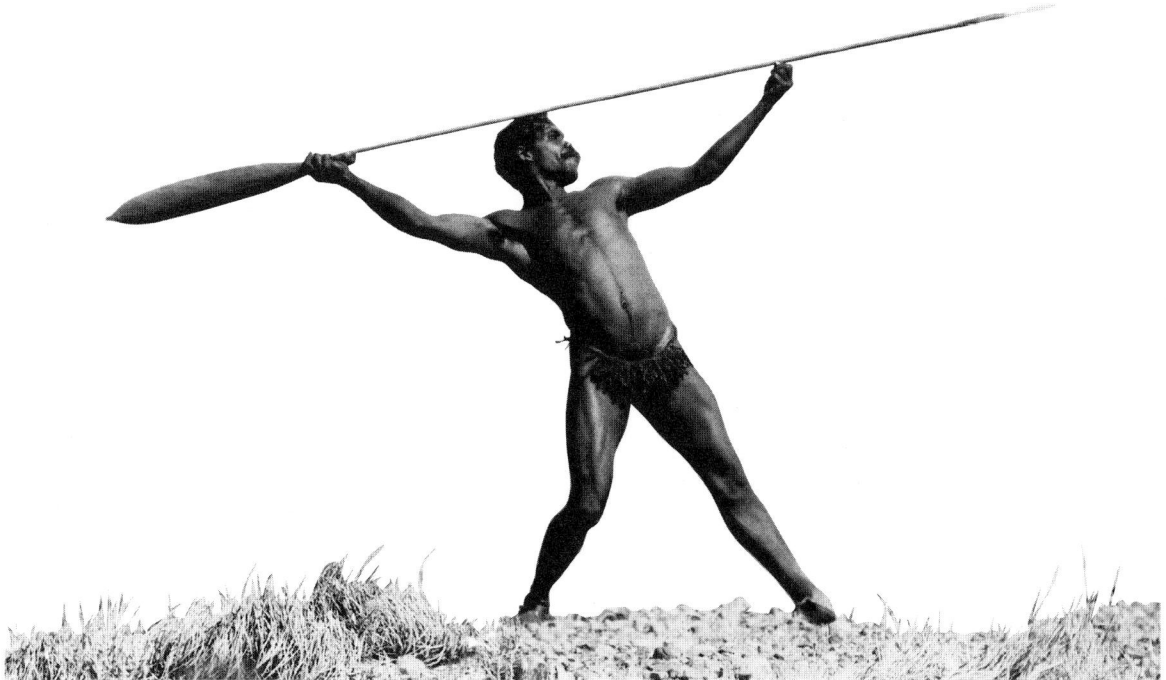

Consider this question

How does each of the sources help you to understand medicine in prehistoric times?

A mark scheme for assessing your answer to Source B might look like this:

Target: Comprehension and inference from an historical source

Level 1: Answer that selects detail (1 mark)
E.g. the painting shows they knew about animals.

Level 2: Answer that draws a simple inference from the source (2–3 marks)
E.g. the painting is probably a man dressed in animal skins so it shows that they had something like a witch doctor.

Level 3: Answer that develops a complex inference from the source (4–5 marks)
E.g. This painting shows a man dressed in animal skins. It shows that people at the time lived close to nature and probably used many natural remedies from plants and animals. This may have been the same in many parts of the world but we can't be sure from just one source.

Now try writing top-level answers for Sources A and C.

✎ Revision Tips

People living in prehistoric society did not have writing. This means that sources used in examinations are likely to be pictures, and questions are likely to be simple.

Make sure you understand what an inference is and how to make one from a source. Look back at page 6 of the Introduction.

Key features of society in the ancient world

Ancient Egypt

Writing and calculating

The Ancient Egyptians were one of the first societies to use these skills. It helped them to record and measure important things for farming, building and running the country. It also helped historians to find out what the Ancient Egyptians did in medicine.

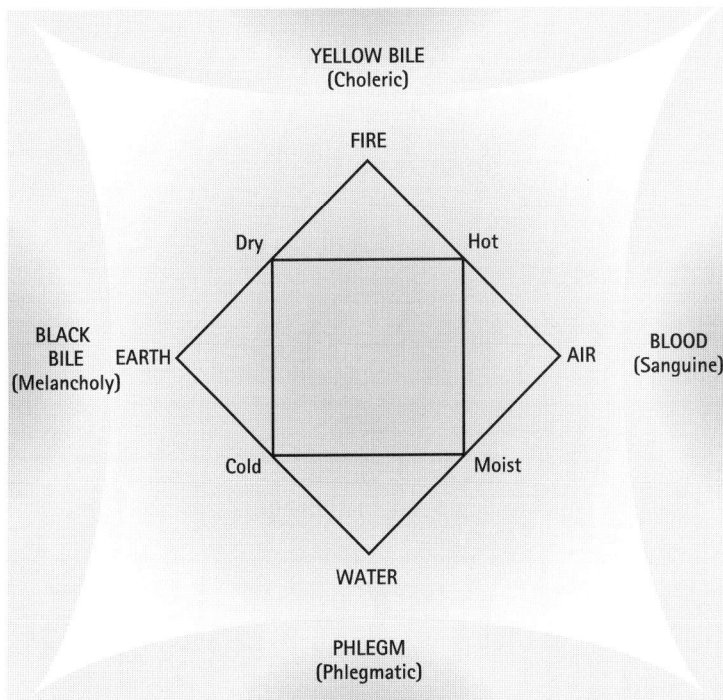

▶ SOURCE D

A cure for burns

Mix milk of a woman who has born a male child with gum and ram's hair. while putting the mixture on the burn say the words of the Goddess Isis, 'My son, Horus is burnt in the desert. Is there any water there? There is no water. I have water in my mouth and a Nile between my thighs. I have come to extinguish the fire.'

Ancient Greece

Logical theories about the natural world

The Ancient Greeks believed in Gods. They also had philosophers such as Aristotle and Hippocrates who believed in logic and mathematics. They were more interested in using natural ideas to explain medicine and health.

◀ SOURCE E

Diagram of the four humours

Ancient Rome

A strong government and a large army

The Ancient Romans conquered Egypt, Greece and many other parts of the world. This gave them knowledge and ideas from all these places. Many of the things they built like baths and aqueducts survive all over the world even today.

People from ancient societies often lived in towns. They developed farming rather than hunting to get food and this allowed people to follow full-time professions like priests and doctors.

▶ SOURCE F

Picture of a Roman aqueduct near Nimes in France

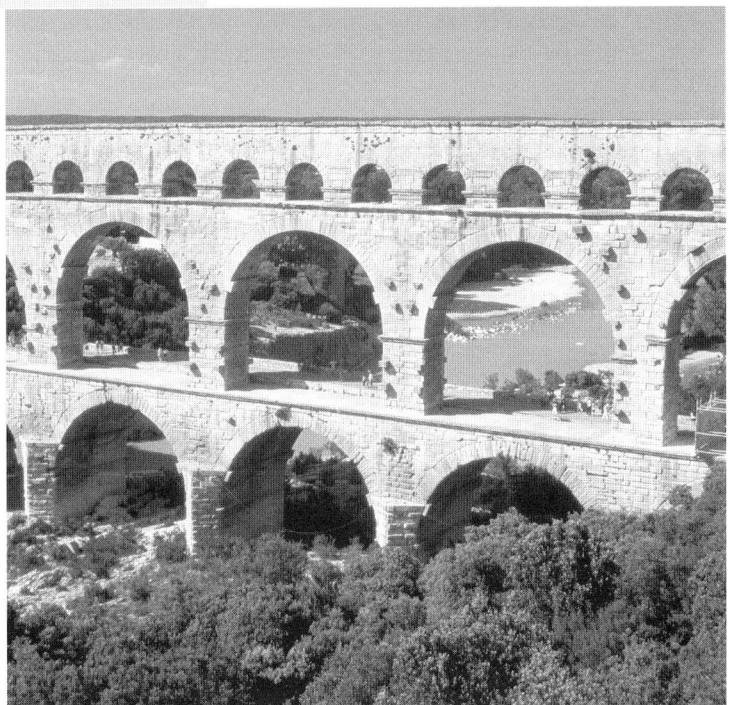

✎ Revision Tips

Using all six sources A to F, the examiner is now in a position to ask you a number of questions about similarities or differences between medical practices at various times or about developments in medicine over time:

- How do the sources show that medicine had changed?
- How do the sources show continuity in ideas about medicine?
- Does Source F show that public health was more important than medicine to the Romans?
- What developments in ideas about medicine are shown by these sources?

Write answers to these questions.

Consider this question

Does Source D show progress in medicine between prehistoric times and the Ancient Egyptian period? Explain your answer using Sources B and D and your own knowledge.

A mark scheme for assessing your answer might look like this:

Target: Identifying change using two historical sources

Level 1: Answer that describes the content (1–2 marks)
> E.g. The Egyptians used a strange mixture to cure burns. In prehistoric times there was nothing they could do.

Level 2: Answer that provides an inference from the source(s) (3–4 marks)
> E.g. The Egyptians made an ointment for the burn and prayed to their god. In prehistoric times they had no practical cure like an ointment.

Level 3: Answer that sets the sources in the context of knowledge (5–6 marks)
> E.g. In prehistoric times we know that magic was used a lot in medicine as shown by Source B, which is probably a witch doctor. At the same time they did use practical treatments like putting a broken leg in a mud plaster until it healed. This was an Aborigine practice used in modern times. This isn't much different from the Egyptian papyrus in Source D. From my own knowledge however I do know that the Egyptians were more civilized and did have proper doctors.

Ancient Greece

✎ Revision Tips

Look carefully at Source G on the next page and compare it with Source E.

What does Source G tell you about developments in medicine made by the Ancient Greeks when you compare it with Source E?

What questions would you ask and how would you answer them?

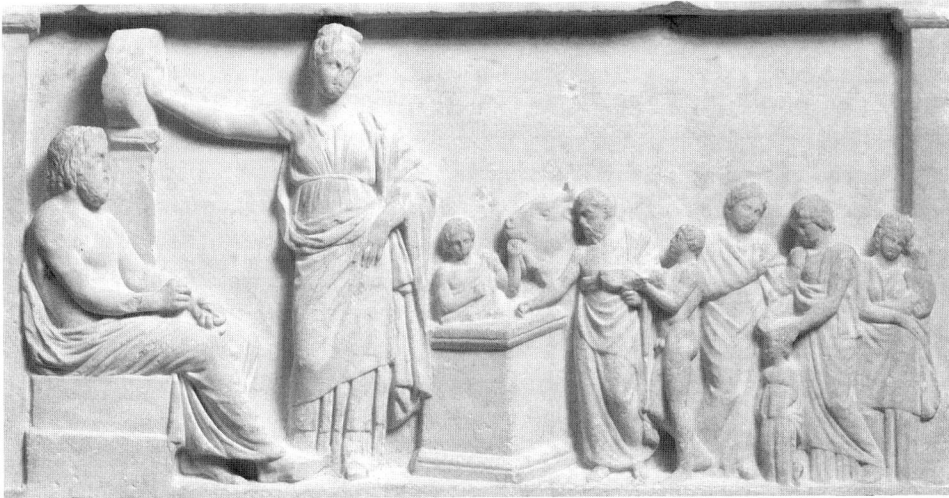

Key features of medicine in the ancient world: Ancient Egypt

Natural theories of how the body worked

The secret knowledge of the heart and the heart's movements:

46 channels go from the heart to every part of the body. If a doctor, a priest of Sekhmet or a magician, places his hand on the head, hands, stomach, arms or feet then he hears the heart. The heart speaks out of every limb. There are four channels in the nose, 2 for mucus, 2 for blood.

There are four channels in the forehead which give blood to the eyes...

▲ SOURCE A

An account of the inside of the body from one of the surviving Egyptian medical books, the Ebirs Papyrus

Supernatural theories of how illness could be caused or cured

▶ SOURCE B

The goddess Sekhmet who Egyptians believed had the power to cure or cause illness

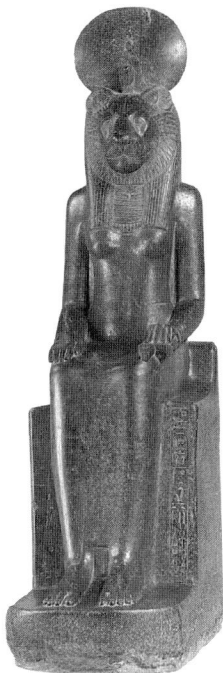

Natural medical or religious reasons?

▼ SOURCE C

Written by the Greek historian, Heredotus, in the fifth century BC

The Egyptian priests shave their whole body every third day so no lice may infect them while they are serving the gods.

Natural medicine from a supernatural doctor?

▼ SOURCE D

The funeral inscription of one of Sekhmet's priests

I was a priest of Sekhmet strong and skilful in the Art: One who put his hands upon the sick and so found out; One who is skilful with his eye.

Revision Tips

Societies like those of Ancient Egypt present a confusing mixture of natural and supernatural medical ideas and treatments. You can see this clearly in Sources A–D. It is likely that exam questions will want you to show that you are aware of this.

In writing answers use your knowledge of the main features of medicine and society such as:

- The importance of the River Nile to Egyptian life and farming and its connection with the ideas shown in Source A.

- The importance of gods and religion in explaining why crops grew and people became ill.
- The role of mummification as a religious not a medical practice.
- The importance of farming and trade in creating wealth and leisure time.
- The connection between wealth, religion and the growing number of professional doctors.
- The existence of natural remedies based on knowledge of plants and experience of their properties.

Key features of medicine in the ancient world: Ancient Greece

Supernatural medicine

▶ SOURCE A

A statue of Asklepios, the god of healing

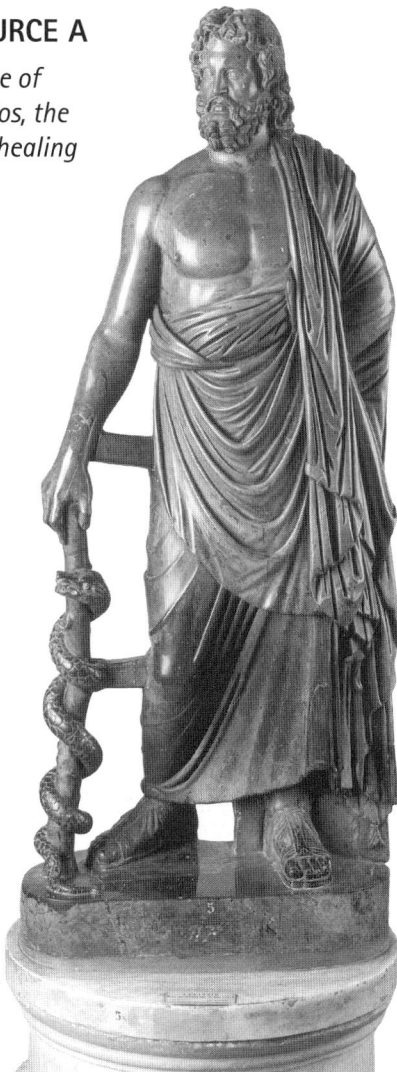

Rational medicine

It is not, in my opinion, any more divine or sacred than other diseases are; there are natural signs. Men believe only that it is a divine disease because of their ignorance....

(*SHP Early Man and Medicine*, (Holmes McDougall, 1976) p30)

▲ SOURCE B
From a Greek book on 'The Sacred Disease' (epilepsy)

Alternative treatment

Despairing of human skill but with all hope in the divine, leaving Athens, blessed in her sons, and coming to your grove, Asklepios, I was cured in three months of a wound in the head that had lasted for a whole year.

▲ SOURCE C
From a poem by the Greek poet, Aischines.

Rational based on supernatural

Part of the Hippocratic oath

I will swear by Apollo, Asklepios and by all the gods that I will carry out this oath. I will use treatment to help the sick according to my ability and judgement but never with a view to injury or wrongdoing. I will not give poison to anybody....

(*SHP Early Man and Medicine*, (Holmes McDougall, 1976) p34)

✎ Revision Tips

A glance at Sources A–D suggests that medicine in Ancient Greece was very much like medicine in Ancient Egypt: a confusing mixture of the natural and supernatural. An examiner could choose sources which show one thing or the other, so always use your knowledge to check which side of the picture a source is giving. Source C gives clues about why Greeks often used both types of medicine. Look back at page 13.

Apart from these sources you should also have knowledge of:

- The life and work of Aristotle (see page 18).
- The life and work of Hippocrates (see page 18).
- The importance of physical fitness and exercise to the Ancient Greeks.
- The importance of Alexandria as a university and library where doctors could dissect human bodies.
- The importance of trade in giving the Greeks contact with ideas from India, China and Egypt.

All these things are factors that helped Greek medicine to change and develop.

Key features of medicine in the ancient world: Ancient Rome

Herbal and natural cures

▶ **SOURCE A**
A remedy written by a Roman politician

If you have reason to fear sickness, give the patient or the oxen the following before they get sick: 3 grains of salt, 3 laurel leaves, 3 spikes of leek, 3 of garlic, 3 grains of incense, 3 plants of Sabine herb, 3 leaves of rue, 3 stalks of byrony, 3 white beans and 3 pints of wine. Administer the medicine to each ox or patient for three days.

Against Greek doctors

▶ **SOURCE B**
From the writings of a Roman military leader

Our ancestors did not condemn healing but they disapproved of medicine as a job. They did not like the idea of making money from saving lives. Of all the Greek sciences, only medicine has not yet gained wide interest among us serious and sober-minded Romans.

Revision Tips

Ancient Roman civilisation covers a long period of time. Rome was founded in about 753 BC when the Greeks and Egyptians were still quite powerful. It did not become the famous Roman Empire until nearly 700 years later at about the time Christ was born. Its power in Europe went into decline about 500 years later. From the point of view of medicine it is useful to think of two periods.

(1) Ancient Rome 700 BC to the birth of Christ and conquest of Britain.

The key features of this society were:

- the importance of farming;
- the growth of trade in the Mediterranean area;
- the conquest of Greece;
- the development of the city of Rome.

The key features of medicine during this early Roman period were:

- family remedies passed down from father to son;
- religious healing centres based on gods like Asklepios;
- commonsense remedies based on plants and herbs;
- hostility to new ideas from well-educated Greek doctors who travelled to Italy.

Consider this question

What do Sources A and B tell you about early Roman medicine?

(2) The Roman Empire from the birth of Christ and the conquest of Britain to the destruction of Rome in about AD 400.

The key features of this period were:

- the growth of the army and the conquest of Europe;
- the building of baths, aqueducts and health facilities all over the empire;
- the growth and adoption of Christianity;
- the increasing use of Greek medicine from Hippocrates;
- the work of Claudius Galen AD 130–201 and other Greek doctors;
- the continued use of herbs and commonsense medicine for ordinary people.

Public Health in Roman Britain

▶ **SOURCE C**

Reconstruction of the outdoor exercise yard and swimming pool at the baths in Wroxeter

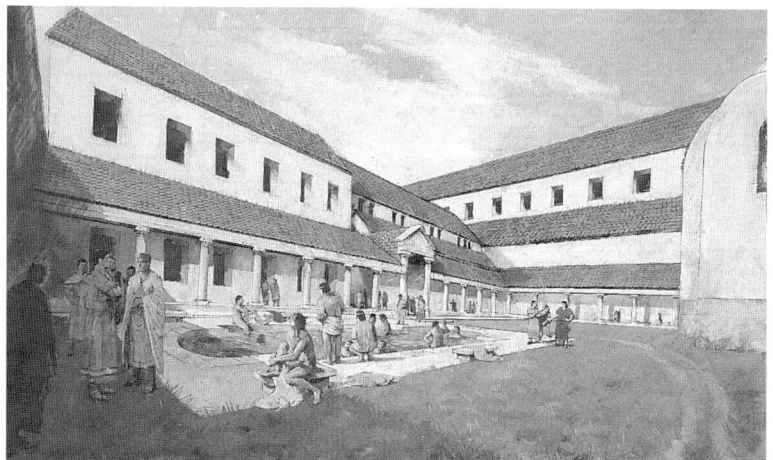

There were bathhouses in most of the Roman towns of Britain.

People of all backgrounds would have been able to use these facilities for a small charge.

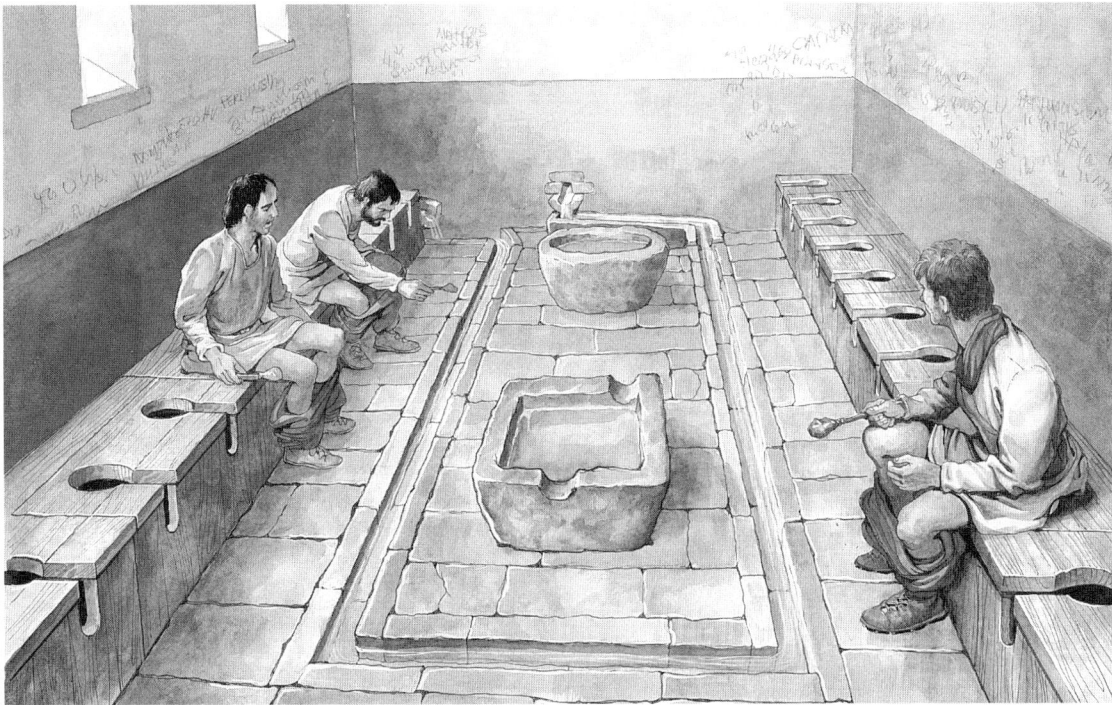

▲ SOURCE D

Reconstruction picture of the legionary latrine at Housesteads on Hadrian's Wall

The Roman Army was important in Britain. Bathhouses and hospitals were built at most army headquarters throughout the country.

Revision Tips

Archaeologists have discovered the remains of Roman public health facilities all over Britain:

- baths, latrines and hospitals along Hadrian's Wall;
- baths at Caerleon in Wales, Chichester, Leicester, Wroxeter;
- a religious healing centre at the baths in Bath;
- underground pipes for sewage in York, Lincoln and Colchester;
- clay pipes coated with concrete to bring fresh water to Lincoln;
- public toilets in St Albans;
- aqueducts in Dorchester and Wroxeter.

There are many more examples of the facilities Romans built in Britain but beware:

- The facilities provided by the Romans were primitive compared with modern sanitation and would often get blocked when the weather was dry;
- There is no evidence of fresh water supply or toilets in most ordinary houses;
- Facilities may only have been built to impress local British rulers so that they would support the invading Romans.

Consider this question

What can you learn from Sources C and D about public health in Roman Britain? Explain your answer using the sources and your own knowledge.

The role of individuals in medical developments in the ancient world

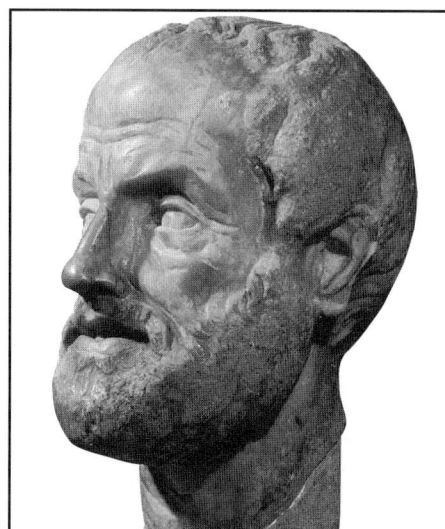

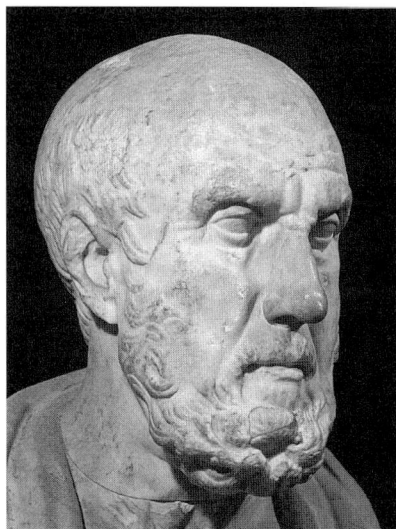

Hippocrates 460–380 BC

The Hippocratic treatises of the fifth century BC refer to many non-drug remedies, such as bloodletting, special diets, baths, exercise or rest, and applications of heat and cold. In addition, more than 300 medications are named, most of plant origin; they could be given by mouth, rectum, vagina, and other orifices. Hippocratic doctors tended to be conservative in their treatment philosophy. They believed in the healing power of nature.

(From *History of Medicine*, Jacalyn Duffin, (Macmillan Press Ltd, 2000))

Key features of his medicine:

* rejection of magic;
* clinical observation;
* the four humours;
* preventative medicine;
* The Hippocratic oath.

Consider this question

How important was the role of Hippocrates in the development of medicine in the ancient world?

Aristotle 384–322 BC

Despite artistic influences and their skill in observation, Greek doctors were not especially interested in anatomy. Dissection of human bodies was forbidden, and funeral practices centred on cremation.

The ban on dissection did not extend to animals. The fourth century BC philosopher and biologist, Aristotle, appears to have used large diagrams when he taught the anatomy of animals. Unfortunately none of the original drawings have survived.

(From *History of Medicine*, Jacalyn Duffin, (Macmillan Press Ltd, 2000))

Key features of his thinking:

* observation of the real world;
* dissection of animals;
* studied and explained connections between the heart, brain and blood vessels.

Galen AD 130–201

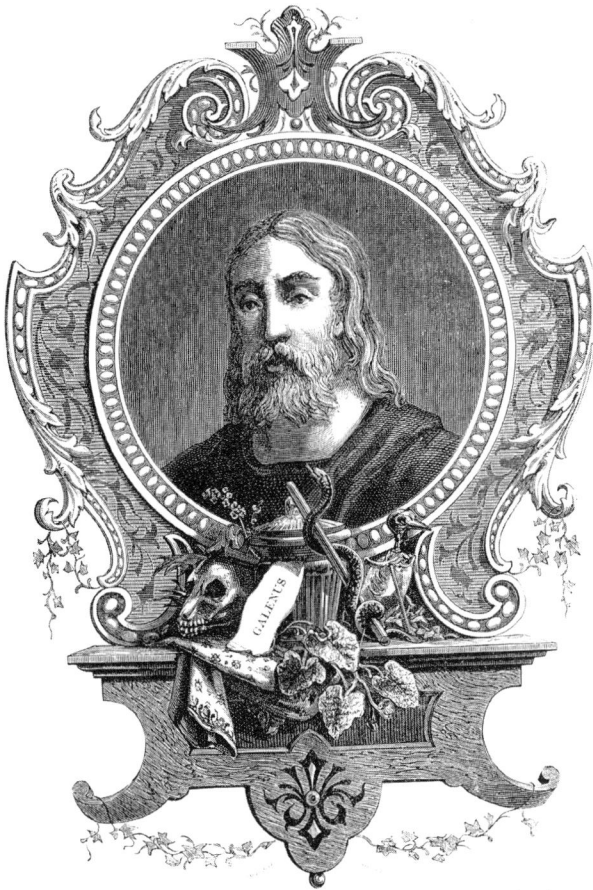

Treating the Emperor

Something really amazing happened the first time I treated the Emperor Marcus Aurelius. Three doctors had watched him since dawn and all three said that a fever was coming. I took his pulse. Far from indicating a fever, the pulse told me that his stomach was stuffed with food, and this had become a slimy excrement. The Emperor praised my diagnosis and said over and over, 'That is it. It is just as you say. I have eaten too much cold food.' He asked what should be done. I replied, 'Usually I prescribe wine with pepper. In this case it will be enough to place a woollen cover over your stomach, soaked in hot spices'.

▲ **SOURCE A**

Galen's books took ideas from:

- India;
- the theory of the four humours;
- human dissection at Alexandria.

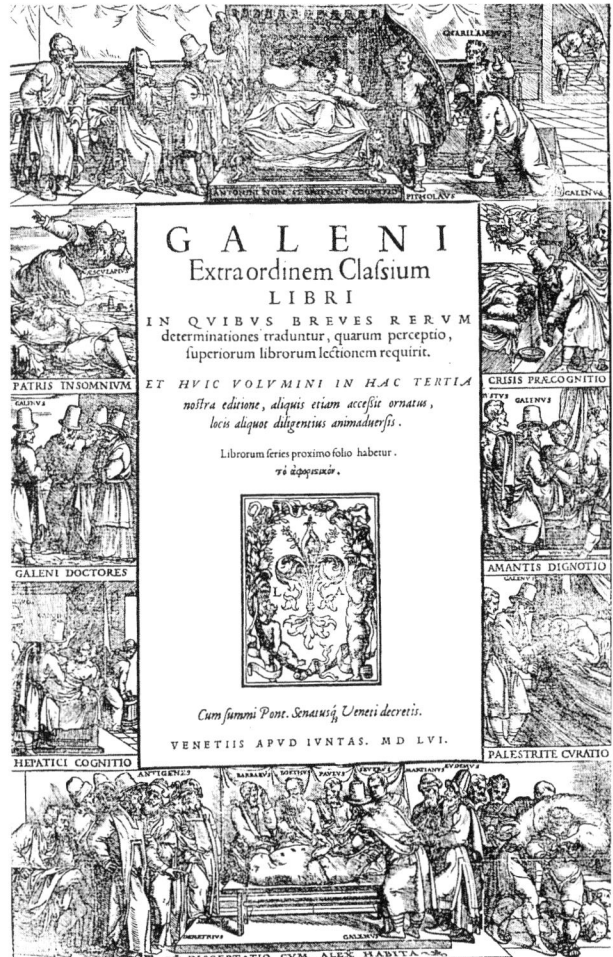

▲ **SOURCE B**

Printed cover of Galen's works

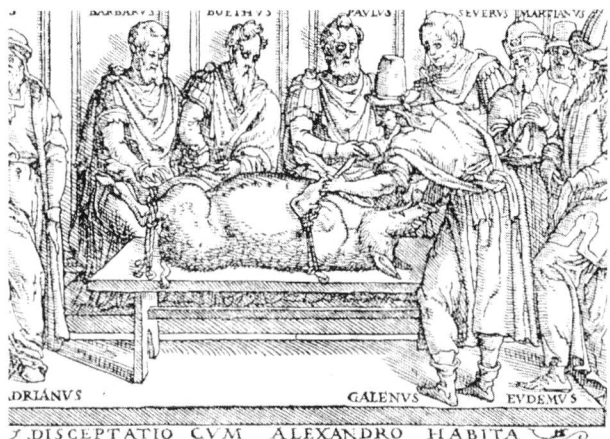

▲ **SOURCE C**

Dissecting a pig

19

Galen became famous in the Roman Empire because:

- he treated famous people successfully; and
- he praised his own work in public.

His writings were respected by doctors in Europe and western Asia for the next 1500 years.

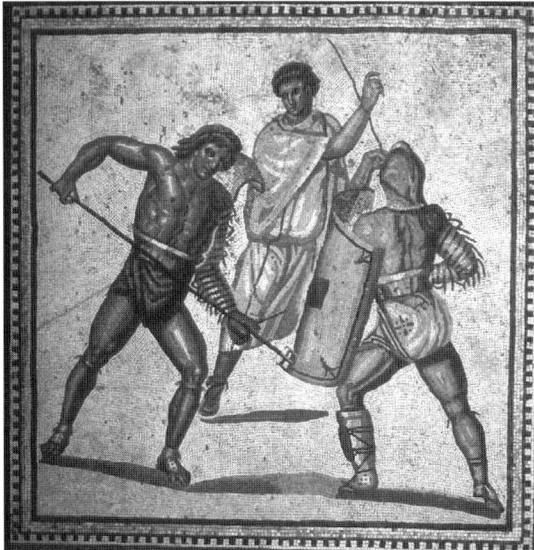

◀ **SOURCE D**

Roman gladiators

What the historical evidence shows about medicine in the ancient world

Examples of questions and answers that might be included in Section B of an examination paper.

✎ Revision Tips

First look back at what you will be expected to answer in Section B. You can find this on page 4 of the Introduction. Think about these key points:

- Each question is likely to have two parts.
- Each question is likely to have one source.

Now review possible questions by looking back through the pages of the book. You will find:

- How does each of the sources help you to understand medicine in prehistoric times? **On page 10.**

This example question covers the sort of thing you might be asked about prehistoric medicine. Other areas of medicine in the ancient world that might be used to set questions are:

- Ancient Egypt;
- the cult of Asklepios;
- the theory of the four humours;

- the library at Alexandria;
- Ancient Rome;
- the development of public health in Rome;
- medicine in the Roman Army;
- the importance of Aristotle;
- the importance of Galen.

Remember that the source question on Section B will be based on one source. Your answers will be marked on two things:

- **Comprehension** or understanding of what the source says or shows.
- **Inference** or your opinion, based on the reasoning you use to explain what you think the source shows or says (look back at page 6 of the Introduction).

Consider the example questions and mark scheme on the next page then try to set some questions of your own to cover the missing areas.

Consider this question

Study Source D on page 11 showing an Ancient Egyptian cure for burns, then look at this question and example mark scheme.

What does Source D tell you about the cures used by the Ancient Egyptians?

A mark scheme for assessing your answer might look like this:

Target: Comprehension and inference from historical source

Level 1: Answer that selects detail

E.g. The Egyptians used strange mixtures and prayed to their gods to cure people. (You should get 1 or 2 out of 3 marks for such an answer.)

Level 2: Answer that draws a simple inference from the source

E.g. The source tells me that the Ancient Egyptians used supernatural cures. (You should get 1 or 2 out of 3 marks for such an answer.)

Comments

You can see that this is a simple question that is not worth many marks and shouldn't take you long to answer.

Consider these questions and write answers for each one.

- What can you learn from Source C (page 10) about medicine in prehistoric times?
- What does Source F (page 11) tell you about the Roman approach to health and medicine?
- Does Source G (page 13) show that Greek medicine was based on supernatural beliefs? Use the source and your knowledge to explain your answer.
- What does Source C (page 13) tell you about hygiene in Ancient Egypt?
- What does Source D (page 13) tell you about medicine in Ancient Greece?

Revision Tips

Remember that medicine in the ancient world was a confusing mixture of supernatural and natural practices. There are no right or wrong answers to the above questions. The examiner will be looking for answers that understand the limits of a single source of evidence and use clear reasoning to explain those limits.

Key features of the development of medicine in the ancient world

The second part of a question in Section B will be much more difficult than the first part. It will go beyond simply looking at a source of evidence and will ask you to use your knowledge of developments in medicine. Your answers will need to use extended writing. You will be asked to explain why things happened or did not happen in one or more of the three main areas of your study. These are:

- cause and cure;
- anatomy and surgery;
- public health.

Revision Tips

Review these points of development by turning them into diagrams with dates and other important details.

Cause and cure of disease:

- the role of plants and magic in prehistoric medicine;
- blocked bodily channels or evil spirits as reasons for disease in Ancient Egypt;
- treatment by visiting an Asklepion or a doctor who uses the four humours in Ancient Greece;
- prevention of disease through public health or visiting a Greek doctor in Ancient Rome.

Anatomy and surgery:

- trephination and practical knowledge of anatomy;
- mummification or knowledge of the body gained from sacrificing animals in Ancient Egypt;
- human dissection in Alexandria;
- the work of Claudius Galen.

Public health:

- nomadic lifestyles in prehistoric societies;
- the development of towns and farming in the ancient world;
- the importance of hygiene and exercise in ancient medical writing;
- government promotion of public health by the Romans.

Revision Tips

When you have constructed your revision diagrams to show the main developments in medicine you can improve them further by thinking about the different things which caused change or held it back. These are often referred to in examinations as factors. The main ones are:

- warfare;
- chance;
- science and technology;
- government and political action;
- the work of specific individuals;
- religion and superstition.

Good answers explain how different factors worked together to encourage or prevent change at different times.

Consider this question

How important was the work of Hippocrates in explaining the cause and cure of disease in the ancient world?

A mark scheme for assessing your answer might look like this:

Target: Assessing the importance of an individual (factor) in medicine

Level 1: Generalised answer (1–3 marks)
E.g. The work of Hippocrates was very important because he used natural ideas to diagnose and treat disease.

Level 2: Developed answer that explains the importance of Hippocrates *or* other factors (4–6 marks)
E.g. Before Hippocrates and the Ancient Greeks most people thought that disease was caused by gods and spirits who were angry, but Hippocrates disagreed with this because he developed the idea of the four humours, which explained disease as something that had natural causes and natural cures. This was a big step forward.

E.g. Hippocrates was not very important because his ideas about the four humours were wrong. Most people, even in Roman times, continued to visit temples such as the Asklepion and rely on the supernatural if they were sick.

Level 3: Developed answer that explains the importance of Hippocrates *and* other factors (7–9 marks)
If you put both the examples in Level 2 together you would get an answer to reach this level.

Level 4: As for Level 3 but with a clearly supported judgement about the importance of Hippocrates (10–12 marks)
All you would have to add to Level 3 would be something like:
E.g. However, Hippocrates' work lasted and was taken up later by people such as Galen, but even though it spread and was a natural theory it was wrong and did not always cure people so they continued to turn to religion or in the case of the Romans to prevention rather than cure.

Comment

There are no tricks here but you need to have good knowledge to reach the top level. There are several important things to remember:

- This is not a question about everything Hippocrates ever did.
- You need to be able to write about other factors causing or preventing developments in medicine apart from the one mentioned in the question.
- You need to plan your answer in the style of levels 2, 3 and 4 of the mark scheme.
- You do not have to get every level in your answer to reach the top level. In this question, a combination of levels 3 and 4 is all that is needed to reach the top.

Consider this question

Why did the Romans believe in preventing rather than curing disease?

A mark scheme for assessing your answer might look like this:

Target: Understanding the reasons for medical ideas and practices

Level 1: Generalised answer (1–3 marks)
E.g. The Romans had a good public health system which nearly everyone was able to use.

Level 2: *Either*
Answer that describes what the Romans did (4–6 marks)
E.g. The Romans believed in prevention rather than cure because they looked after their people by not building towns near unhealthy marshes, providing clean water from the mountains by aqueducts, taking waste away in sewers and providing public baths and toilets. This worked, so they believed in it.

Or

Answer that explains one cause in detail (4–6 marks)
E.g. They believed in prevention rather than cure because most of the cures didn't work. They were based on the four humours practised by foreign Greek doctors who charged a lot of money for these poor treatments.

Or

Answer that simply lists a lot of different causes (4–6 marks)
E.g. The Romans believed in this because they did not trust doctors, they were practical people, they needed to keep the army healthy and they were good at building.

Level 3: Answer that explains several different reasons in some detail such as the middle one in Level 2 (7–9 marks)

Level 4: Answer like Level 3, but it will give details and link the different reasons together or explain which was the most important reason and why (10–12 marks)

Comment

'Why' questions look much easier than 'how important' questions, but as you can see you still need to:

- write about different reasons to reach the top level;
- plan your answer carefully to show links and explanations.

The development of medicine in the ancient world. What do you think?

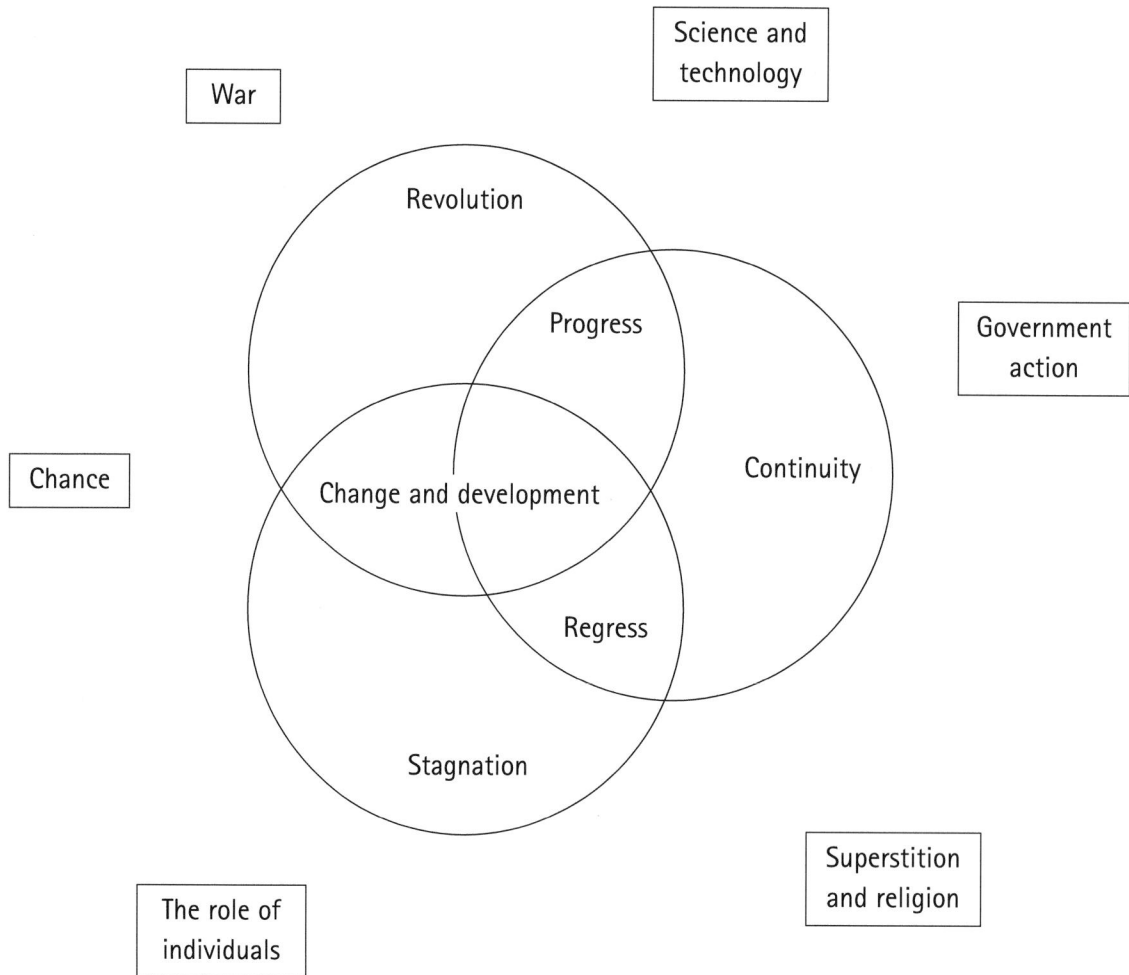

Science and technology

War

Revolution

Progress

Government action

Chance

Change and development

Continuity

Regress

Stagnation

Superstition and religion

The role of individuals

✎ **Revision Tips**

Make your own circle diagram on a large piece of paper.

- Cut out your words and circles, then link them together for different times such as prehistoric, Egypt, Greece and Rome.
- Find examples of the factors for that time.
- Stick or write them onto the circle in the place you think is most relevant for that time.

2. Medicine in the Medieval and Renaissance World

A summary of what you need to know about the medieval and Renaissance world

Exam Paper	Sections A and B	Sections A and B	Section C
Theme Time	Cause, prevention and cure of disease	Practices of anatomy and surgery	Public health in Britain
AD 500 The Dark Ages	Impact of the fall of the Roman Empire on medicine	Impact of the fall of the Roman Empire on medicine	Impact of the fall of the Roman Empire on public health in Britain
AD 700 The early Middle Ages	Islamic empire established Hospital in Baghdad and centre of learning		Saxon and Viking invasions
	Impact of superstition and Christianity on European medicine	Continued reliance on the works of Hippocrates and Galen	Monasteries established throughout Britain and Europe
AD 1000	Rhazes Ibn Sina (Avicenna)	Religious hospitals set up throughout Europe	
AD 1300 The later Middle Ages	Baghdad destroyed by invading Mongols		
			The Black Death
AD 1500 The European Renaissance	Paracelsus	Andreas Vesalius Ambroise Pare William Harvey	
AD 1700			The Great Plague

✎ Revision Tips

The Middle Ages and Renaissance cover a long period of time. Break it down into shorter periods:

- Early Middle Ages or 'Dark Ages' from AD 500–1200 when Europe was ravaged by war but the Middle East or Islamic empire was making great progress in science and medicine.
- The later Middle Ages from AD 1200–1500 when the Christian Church controlled most of the learning in Europe.
- The Renaissance AD 1500–1700 when the Church began to lose control and individuals challenged old medical ideas.

Key features of early medieval society

The impact of the fall of the Roman Empire

▶ **SOURCE A**
From an Anglo-Saxon poem known as 'The Ruin'

Wondrous is this masonry, shattered by the Fates. The buildings raised by giants are crumbling. The roofs have collapsed, the towers are in ruins. Here were splendid palaces and many halls with water flowing through them. And now these rooms lie desolate. Here stood courts of stone, and a stream gushed forth in rippling floods of hot water.

The impact of superstition and Christian religion

▶ **SOURCE B**
Written by Bede, an Anglo-Saxon writer in the eighth century

When the bishop learned that blood-letting had taken place on the fourth day of the moon he said, 'You have acted most foolishly. Don't you know that it is dangerous to bleed people when the light of the moon and the pull of the tide is increasing?' He went to see the girl and said a prayer over her and left. The girl made a complete recovery.

✎ Revision Tips

The early Middle Ages was very similar to the ancient world in many ways:

- religion was very important;
- there were towns and villages;
- farming was the most important occupation;
- writing was used but only by a small number of educated people;
- there were many wars.

But there were some important differences:

- there was no strong government in Europe like there had been under the Romans;
- the Christian and Islamic Churches were more powerful than most governments;
- many Greek and Roman medical books were lost to Western Europe or preserved only in monasteries;
- Greek and Roman writings found their way into Islamic centres of learning such as Baghdad.

Consider this question

How does Source B help you to understand medicine in the early Middle Ages?

Look back at the ancient world, page 10, then write a Level 3 answer to this question.

✎ Revision Tips

Remember these points:

- Your answer must be based on what the source says.
- You need to explain what the source is telling you about medicine at the time rather than just copy out passages.
- You need to make an **inference**. This means that you have to put forward an idea or

conclusion that comes directly from the source or information. This is more than just picking out details from the source.

- Look back at the mark scheme on page 6 of the Introduction to get an example of how to make an inference. Look at other example questions later in the book as well.

▶ **SOURCE C**

The first description of smallpox, from a book by Rhazes, written in the ninth century.

The outbreak of smallpox begins with continued fever, pain in the back, itching in the nose and terrors in the sleep. These are the specific symptoms of its start:

- a pain in the back with fever;
- a pricking which the patient feels all over the body;
- an inflamed colour and vivid redness in both cheeks;
- redness of both the eyes;
- heaviness of the whole body;
- nausea and anxiety.

The impact of Islamic religion

When Baghdad was destroyed by Mongols in AD 1285 Islamic medical ideas were not lost. They found their way into Europe with religious scholars, traders and crusaders. Many of the ideas were translated into Latin and copied by monks in monasteries. They were taught to European doctors in medical schools set up in places like Bologna in Italy and Montpellier in France. The Church controlled most of the universities, hospitals and monasteries.

What the historical evidence shows about medicine in the medieval world

Examples of questions and answers that might be included in Section A of an examination paper. The specified aspect of medicine through time for 2004 is 'The impact of religion on medicine in the Middle Ages'.

Consider this question

How does Source C show that Islamic religion had a different effect on medical ideas from Christian religion in the early middle ages?

Explain your answer using Sources B and C and your own knowledge.

This is the kind of question you might find on Section A of the paper. It is much more difficult than the question on page 26 because you cannot rely just on the sources. You have to use knowledge to reach the higher levels.

A mark scheme for assessing your answer might look like this:

Target: Identifying differences using two historical sources

Level 1: Answer that describes the content (1–2 marks)
E.g. Source C describes the symptoms of smallpox but Source B talks about a bishop praying to cure a girl.

Level 2: Answer that provides an inference from the source(s) (3–4 marks)
E.g. Rhazes is using observation that shows natural medicine but the Christian bishop is talking about astrology and praying, which shows superstition.

Level 3: Answer that sets the sources in the context of knowledge (5–6 marks)
E.g. When the Roman Empire fell, many of the works of Hippocrates and Galen were lost in Western Europe. As the Christian Church became more powerful it took over medicine and said that disease was caused and cured by God as shown in Source B. In the Islamic world the ideas of the Ancient Greeks were preserved in places like Baghdad so they continued to use observation and natural ideas like those in Source C.

Key features of medicine in the early medieval world

Islamic Medicine

▼ SOURCE D

Scene from an open-air pharmacy taken from a late medieval Middle-Eastern medical book

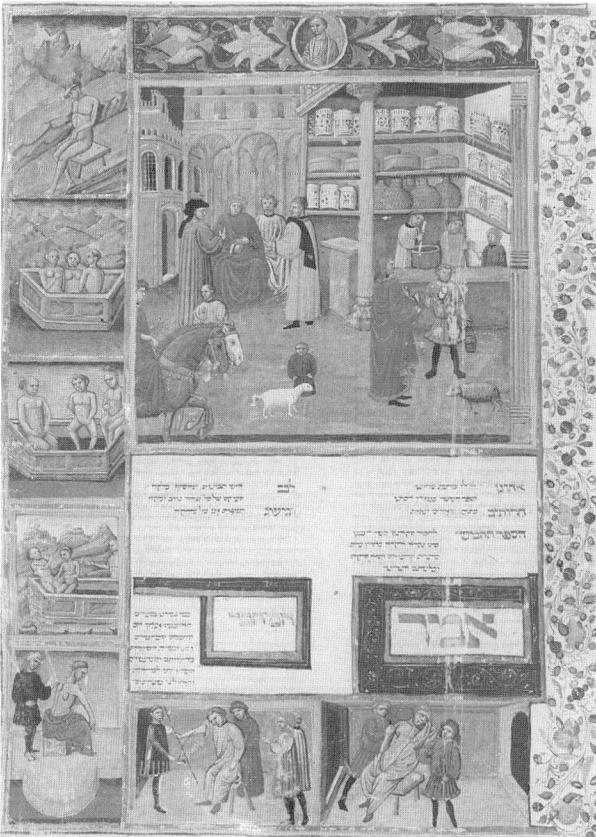

The spread of Islamic medicine

▼ SOURCE E

A late medieval manuscript showing a page from the works of Avicenna used by teachers in England

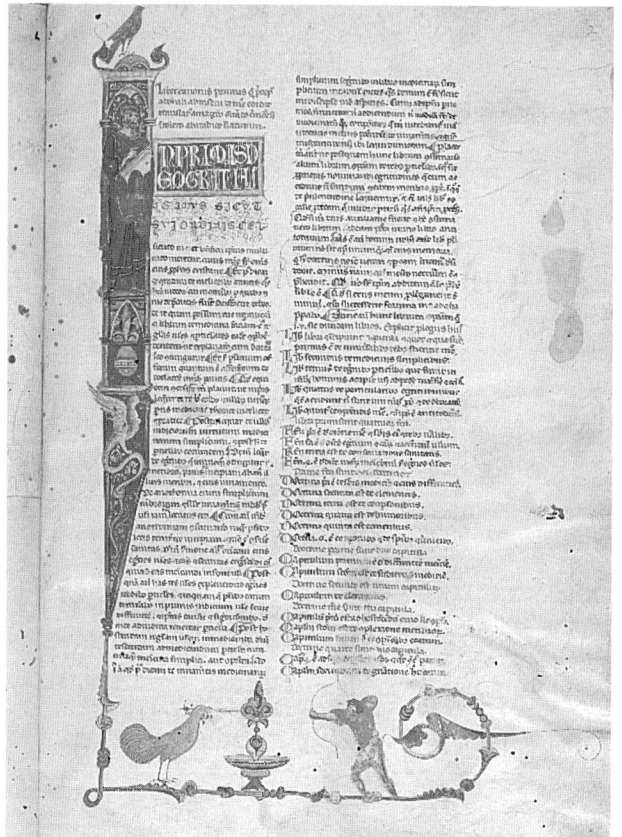

Christian miracles

▼ SOURCE F

*A painting showing saints helped by angels
miraculously replacing a sick white man's leg with the
leg from a dead black man*

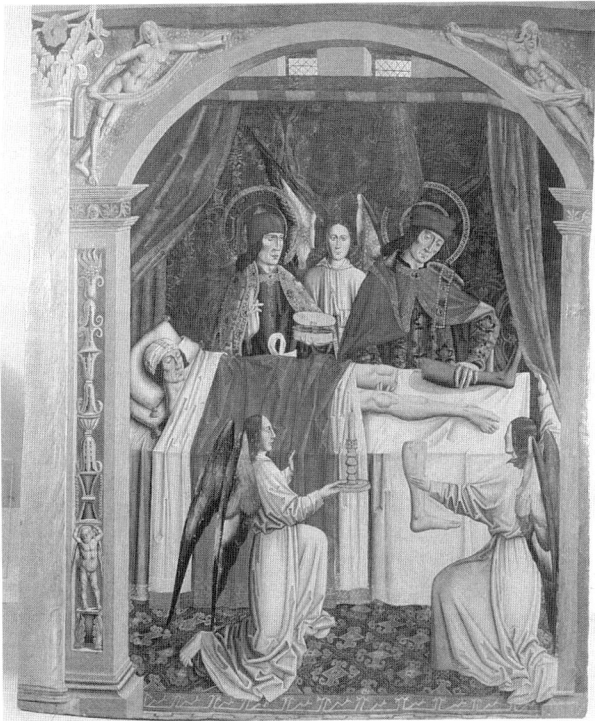

The importance of monasteries

▼ SOURCE G

*Pages from a medical text drawn by an English monk in the eleventh century
showing the use of herbs in treating medical complaints*

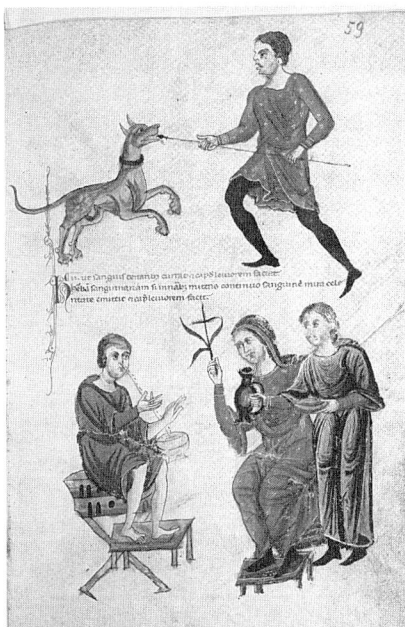

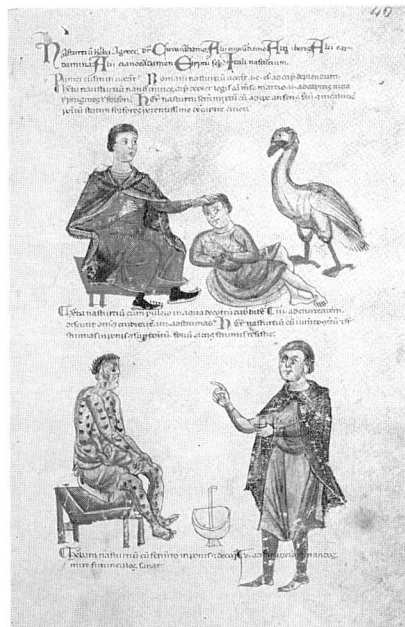

Consider this question

Read the following extract adapted from *Medicine through Time*, a school textbook written by Joe Scott in 1990, and then answer the question that follows.

The Christian Church taught that it was part of people's religious duty to care for the sick but until 1200 it did little to help in the study of medicine.

Study Sources D, E, F and G. **Use the sources and your own knowledge** to explain why you agree or disagree with this interpretation.

A mark scheme for assessing your answer might look like this:

Target: Evaluating an interpretation of the past

Level 1: *Either*

A basic answer that extracts information from sources to agree or disagree
Or

Answer that makes general or undeveloped statements from knowledge (1–3 marks)

Level 2: *Either*

Basic answer that extracts information from sources *and* own knowledge
Or

Answer that develops one or more points using sources *or* knowledge (4–8 marks)

Level 3: Answer that develops one or more points using sources *and* own knowledge (9–12 marks)

Level 4: Developed answer that assesses the interpretation using sources and knowledge to reach a judgement (13–15 marks)

Examiner's comments and level	A top-level answer might look like this:
Extracting information from a source to agree (Level 1)	<u>I think this is true because Source F shows angels sticking a black man's leg on a white man.</u> If they believed that, they knew nothing about medicine so I agree with the interpretation.
Basic answer using knowledge and sources (Level 2)	<u>The Christian Church didn't really help in the study of medicine. The Church told people only to care for and pray for the sick.</u> The monks did keep alive ideas about using herbs and about Hippocrates and Galen, which were translated into Latin.
Developing a point using sources and own knowledge (Level 3)	Sources D and E show Islamic medicine. The Islamic Empire had a strong government and set up a centre of learning in Baghdad. Hospitals were also built that treated all people. In Europe after the fall of the Roman Empire there was chaos and the ideas of Galen and Hippocrates were lost to most people, except in monasteries that were set in secluded areas. <u>If doctors wanted to study medicine they would have to go to an Arab university.</u>
Developed answer which uses sources and knowledge to reach a judgement (Level 4)	There is no doubt that the Church did care for the sick in hospitals and monasteries and in line with what the Bible taught, but it also had the power to stop new ideas about medicine. <u>It made doctors follow the ideas of Hippocrates and Galen. The interpretation is from a school textbook so the author might have wanted to simplify the role of the Church before 1200. Monks may have studied medicine but on balance I would agree with the interpretation.</u>

The role of the Church in medieval medicine is complicated. Study it carefully.

Comments

Section A questions on interpretations are important questions. They will usually carry more marks than any other single question on the paper. So think about these things before you answer.

- An interpretation is just one person's point of view based only on the evidence/sources they have looked at.

- If you look carefully at the sources you should nearly always be able to see another interpretation.
- If you cannot find another interpretation in the sources, you should be able to find it from your studies.
- Your answer will be in the form of extended writing so take some time to plan it.
- Look carefully at the mark scheme on page 30. You should be able to use this to make a plan for all questions about interpretations.

✎ Revision Tips

Some points to consider when answering Section A 'source and interpretation questions'.

- **Who wrote or made the source?** *(Author/Purpose knowledge)*

  This might help to explain how accurate it is or why it is different from another source.

  E.g. If it is a male doctor writing about women in medicine during the Middle Ages you might expect him to be against what they did.

  Or

  If it is a Roman writing about Greek doctors in Rome you might expect him to be against what they did.

- **Who was the source written or made for?** *(Audience/Purpose knowledge)*

  This might help to explain how useful it is and what its limitations are.

  E.g. A letter written to a king might be trying to sell him something and may be exaggerated.

  Or

  A schoolbook for young children might be very simple.

  Or

  A book written by a doctor might exaggerate the importance of his own treatments.

- **When was the source written or made?** *(Time of creation knowledge)*

  This might help to explain how useful it is or why it is different from another source.

  E.g. A medieval manuscript on the work of Avicenna used by English doctors in the late Middle Ages might be different from a book written by Avicenna on the same subject in the early Middle Ages.

- **What are you trying to find out from the source(s)?** *(Your purpose)*

  This might help you to explain the limitations and usefulness of sources.

  E.g. Source E on page 28 tells us that Islamic ideas had spread to England by the late Middle Ages, but it does not tell us what those ideas were.

Always read the sources carefully and make sure you answer the question.

Key Features of public health in medieval Britain

Look back at pages 16–17 of the chapter on the Ancient World.

Revisit the **Revision Tips** on Roman public health facilities in Britain. Remember that although there is plenty of evidence of Roman facilities it is not certain how widespread the use of these facilities was by the population of Britain in Roman times.

✎ Revision Tips

Many people in medieval Britain died from infections and diseases. The first great plague came in 1348 (Black Death) and the last one in 1665 (Great Plague). These killed thousands of people very quickly. Just as deadly were the fevers, sickness, diarrhoea and infections, which thousands died from every year.

When thinking about the causes of these public health problems consider:

- the impact of the fall of the Roman Empire on public health in Britain;
- lack of facilities such as baths, toilets and clean water;
- failure of local and central governments to provide and organise facilities;
- ignorance of what really caused disease and infection;
- the role of the Christian Church in explaining plague and disease.

Government action on public health 1

▼ SOURCE A

An order issued by King Edward III in April 1349

> **To the Lord Mayor of London**
>
> Order to cause the human faeces and other filth lying in the streets and lanes in the city to be removed with all speed to places far distant ... and to cause the city and suburbs to be cleaned from all odour so that no great cause of mortality may arise from such smells.

Personal hygiene in the Middle Ages

▼ SOURCE B

A medieval stained glass window showing a woman bathing

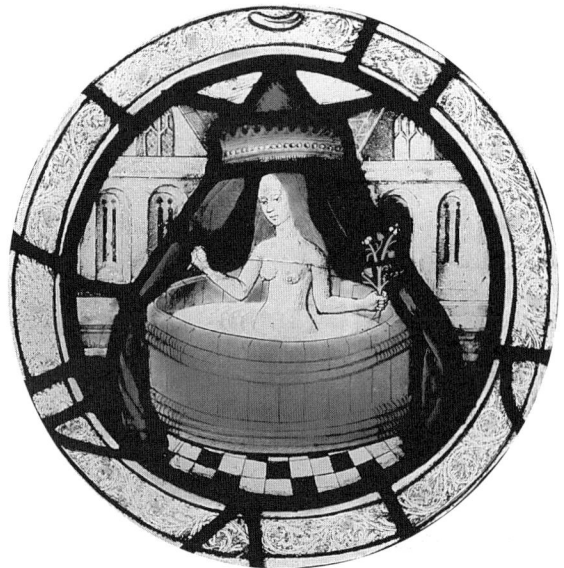

Hygiene in medieval monasteries

▼ SOURCE C

A plan of Canterbury Cathedral Priory in 1160 showing its watercourses

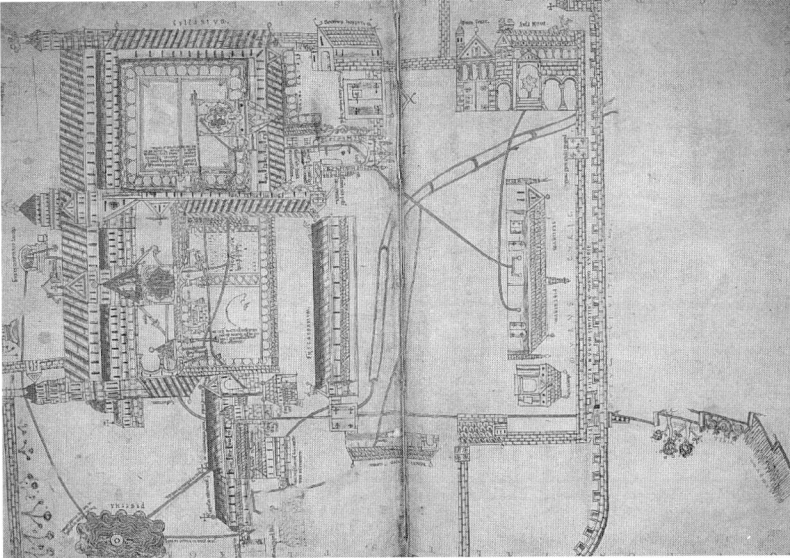

Government action on public health 2

▶ SOURCE D

Regulations issued by the City of London Council in 1665

- Examiners and searchers should be appointed whose job it is to identify houses where the plague has struck and board the houses up to stop the spread of infection
- The dead are only to be buried at night
- Stray dogs are to be killed by council dog killers. No other animals should be kept in the city.

✎ Revision Tips

Section C covers public health in Britain. It will usually have two questions. You will have to **answer only one of these questions**. Each question will have three parts and one source. Only one part of each question will be based on the source. This means that for the other two parts of the question you will be depending on your knowledge of the topic.

Consider this question

What can you learn from Source A about government action on public health in towns and cities in the Middle Ages?

Explain your answer **using Source A and your own knowledge. (5 marks)**

Examiner's comments and level	A top-level answer might look like this:
Knowledge but no mark until candidate makes direct reference to the source	Source A shows that government action on public health in London in 1349 was very poor. <u>This was the time of the Black Death when people were dying in thousands.</u>
Simple inference from the source (Level 2)	<u>If the government had done something then the King would not be ordering them to clean up the streets.</u> We don't even know if the government did what the King told them.
Candidate sets the source in the context of knowledge (Level 3)	Even if they <u>did it wouldn't help much because the Black Death was not caused by bad smells but by germs carried by fleas on rats.</u> They didn't know this at the time. This was in London.
Simple evaluation of source for limitation, not rewarded in the mark scheme	<u>We don't know what was happening in other towns and cities because this is only a source about London.</u>

Comment

This example, and the one on page 30, shows you how examiners mark your answers. Most questions have a mark scheme with three or four levels.

The examiners will mark on your answer paper where you have achieved a particular level, usually by underlining the relevant words. They will then write the level on the left-hand side with any comment they wish to make. The mark awarded will be shown on the right-hand side.

The target for this question would be: Comprehension and inference from an historical source.

Notice that a display of knowledge cannot be rewarded unless the source is also used or referred to. Simple evaluation is also not rewarded. **You must answer the question.**

Consider this question

Did public health in Britain get worse during the Middle Ages? Explain your answer.

A mark scheme for assessing your answer might look like this:

Target: Understanding the concept of regression

Level 1: Generalised answer (1–3 marks)
E.g. Yes because people began to throw all their rubbish in the streets. They had no proper toilets or clean water, so Britain became a dump.

Level 2: *Either*
Developed answer that agrees (4–6 marks)
E.g. Before the Middle Ages the Romans had set up public health in Britain. They had built public baths in the main cities, which were cheap enough for most people to use. They had also brought their ideas about clean water and public toilets. When Rome was destroyed, Britain was invaded by barbarians who did not have the time or interest to keep up these facilities. Some of them were frightened by stories of Roman ghosts. The facilities went into

decline in the Middle Ages. Small towns and cities grew up but governments were not strong enough to collect taxes to build public health facilities, so public health got worse and plague spread.

Or

Developed answer that disagrees (4–6 marks)
E.g. Public health was not very good in the Dark Ages after the Romans left Britain, but it did gradually get better for many people. Because of the plague outbreaks, city governments did try to clean the streets up and quarantine people who caught the plague. In monasteries they developed good systems for bringing clean water and flushing toilets, and rich people bathed regularly. It wasn't good for everyone but things did not generally get worse.

Level 3: Developed answer that agrees and disagrees (7–9 marks)
Both Level 2 examples in the same answer.

Level 4: As Level 3, but also gives a direct and well-supported judgement (10–12 marks)

Write a top-level answer to this question. When you have written it, mark it like the examples on pages 30 and 34.

Comment
Remember that your answer does not have to include all levels to reach the top. Level 3 and 4 for this question are enough to produce a top-level mark.

The role of individuals in medical developments in medieval and Renaissance times

The Islamic empire

Al-Razi known in Europe as Rhazes (AD 864–935)

- Persian scientist and writer.
- Stressed careful observation.
- First director of a new hospital in Bahdad.
- Recommended building the hospital where meat decayed the least.
- Observed and recorded the difference between smallpox and measles for the first time.

Ibn Sina known in Europe as Avicenna (AD 980–1037)

- Persian doctor and writer.
- Summarised the whole of medical knowledge in his book *The Canon*.
- Included the ideas of Hippocrates and Galen.
- Listed the medical properties of 760 different drugs.

✎ Revision Tips

The work of these two individuals was a very important factor in the development of medicine in the Middle East. It is important to remember, however, that there were other factors that help to explain these developments:

- Individuals were supported by a strong Islamic government.
- The Islamic Empire covered the Middle East, North Africa and parts of Southern Spain. It was a large area.

- The rulers of the empire were actively interested in science and medicine.
- The rulers set up a centre for the translation of Greek manuscripts in Baghdad, which preserved the works of Galen and Hippocrates.

You need to note that all this happened at the same time as most of Europe was just beginning to come out of the Dark Ages.

Now look back at the question on page 27 and see if you can improve your answer by adding more factual details.

The roles of individuals in medical developments in late medieval and Renaissance times

The European Renaissance

Paracelsus (1490–1541)

- Qualified as a doctor in Vienna and gained further qualifications at several Italian universities.
- Travelled widely throughout Europe.
- Publicly burned the works of Galen and Avicenna.
- Treated and healed many important people but upset authorities with his unusual methods and outspoken opposition to their rules.
- Based his healing on philosophy, astronomy, alchemy and wisdom.
- Wrote many of his ideas down on manuscripts but never organised and published them.

Challenging the authority of other doctors

The best of our popular physicians are the ones who do the least harm. But unfortunately some poison their patients with mercury, and others purge or bleed them to death. There are some who have learned so much that their learning has driven out all common sense, and there are others who care a great deal more for their own profit than for the health of their patients

▲ SOURCE A

From Paracelsus-Selected Writings *(Routledge and Kegan Paul, 1951)*

Ambroise Pare 1510–1590

- Trained as a barber–surgeon at the Paris hospital of Hotel Dieu.
- Joined the French army as a military surgeon.
- Became surgeon to the King of France.
- Developed a less painful and more effective treatment for infection from gunshot wounds using an antiseptic ointment rather than a red hot cautery or boiling oil.
- Developed the use of ligatures to stop bleeding rather than a red hot cautery.
- Published his ideas on surgery.

Challenging the practices of other surgeons

▼ SOURCE B

Diagram of an artificial hand designed by Pare for injured soldiers

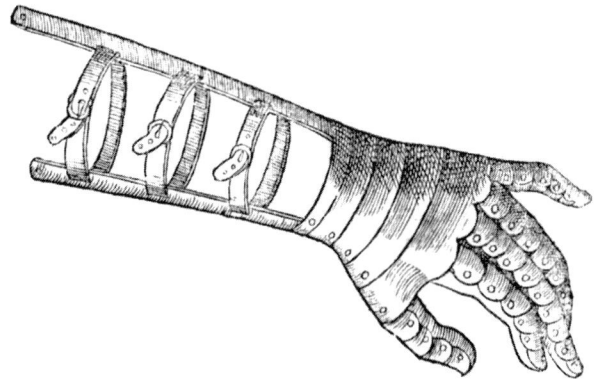

Andreas Vesalius (1514–1564)

- Studied medicine at Louvain, Montpellier and Paris Universities.
- Robbed the body of an executed criminal to study.
- Became Professor of Medicine at Padua when he was only 23.
- Carried out many human dissections and noticed that Galen was wrong about several things, such as the human lower jaw.
- Published the *Fabric of the Human Body* in 1543. It contained many pictures and illustrations by an artist called Jan van Calcar.
- Taught that anatomy should be based on observation not words in old books.
- Showed that the septum of the heart is not porous as Galen had said.

New ideas on anatomy

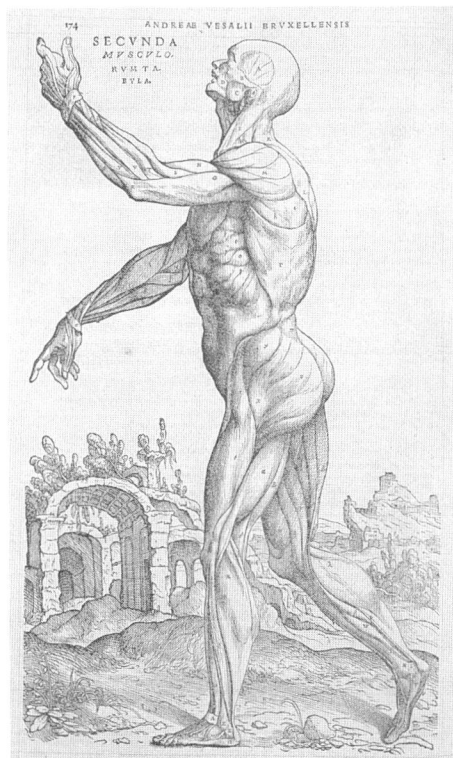

▲ SOURCE C

Illustration from the Fabric of the Human Body *published in 1543*

The Renaissance was a time of great change. It came at the end of the Middle Ages. Artists and scholars became interested in what the Greeks and Romans had done. They followed their methods of looking closely at nature, using first-hand observation not ideas passed down in books. They discovered things that the Greeks and Romans never dreamed of. They questioned accepted practices and ideas such as those of Galen.

William Harvey (1578–1657)

- Worked on human physiology using scientific experiments and careful observation.
- Rejected Galen's ideas that the veins carried blood and air and that blood was absorbed by the body.
- Proved that blood circulated round the body continuously.
- Published a book about the circulation of blood in 1628.

New ideas on physiology

▶ **SOURCE D**

Illustration from Harvey's book on the circulation of blood published in 1628

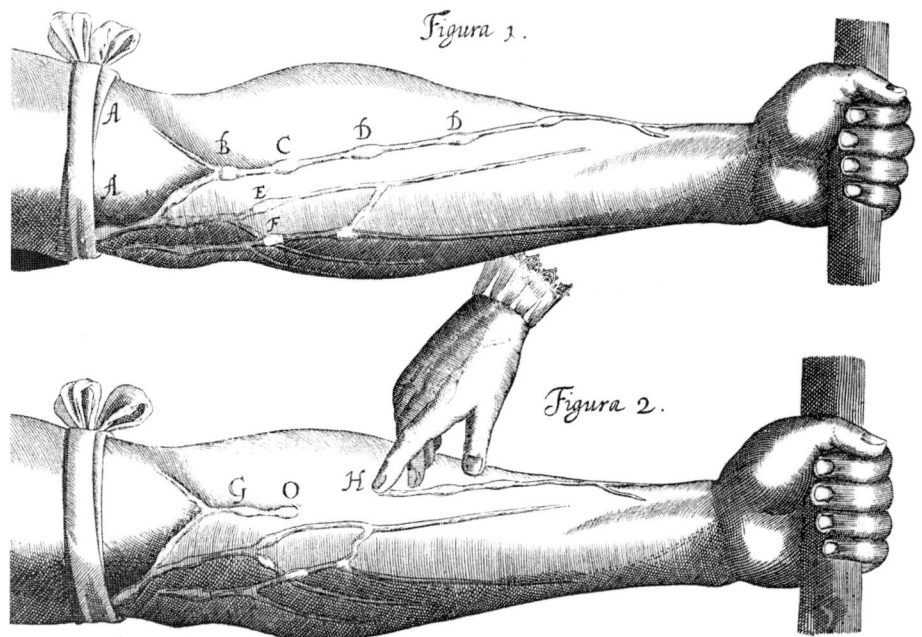

✎ Revision Tips

The work of individuals was only one reason (factor) in explaining why there were great changes in medicine at the time of the **Renaissance**. Other reasons are:

- the discovery of America in 1492 which brought new ideas, plants and products to Europe;
- the invention of printing in Europe in the fifteenth century, which made it easier to copy books and spread ideas;

- the increase in scientific research, which challenged Greek and Roman ideas about the world;
- the decline in the power of the Christian Church which made it easier to spread new ideas without fear of punishment;
- the importance of warfare and the introduction of gunpowder in the improvement of surgery.

A note on human dissection

This remained difficult throughout the Renaissance because doctors could not see its relevance to medicine, and ordinary people were revolted by it.

A French writer in 1788 said:

Anatomy may cure a sword wound, but will prove powerless when the invisible dart of a particular miasma has penetrated beneath our skin.

(Louis Sebastien Mercier in *History of Medicine*, Jacalyn Duffin, (Macmillan Press Ltd, 2000))

✎ Revision Tips

Section B of the examination covers changing ideas and practices in medicine over the whole period of the study. It is the section where you are most likely to be asked about the work of individuals in the Renaissance.

Consider this question

How important was the work of Renaissance individuals in bringing about progress in medicine by 1700? Support your answer with reasons and examples.

A mark scheme for assessing your answer might look like this:

Target: Assessing the importance of a factor in medicine

Level 1: Generalised answer (1–3 marks)

Level 2: Developed answer that explains the importance of individual(s) *or* other factors (4–6 marks)

Level 3: Developed answer that explains the importance of individual(s) *and* other factors (7–9 marks)

Level 4: As Level 3 but with a direct judgement that is well supported (10–12 marks)

Examiner's comments and level	A top-level answer might look like this:
Generalised (Level 1)	<u>Individuals were very important in the Renaissance. People like Vesalius found out a lot about the human body.</u>
Developed importance of individual (Level 2)	<u>Vesalius was a professor at Padua University and while he was there he performed human dissections that proved Galen wrong about the human jaw bone and about the septum being porous. These discoveries were published in 1543 in a book called the *Fabric of the Human Body.* This helped other doctors to test Galen's ideas and come up with new ones like Harvey and the circulation of blood.</u>
Developed other factors (Level 3)	The work of individuals like Vesalius and Harvey was not the only reason progress in medicine was made at this time. <u>The power of the Christian Church was also on the decline and the invention of printing allowed individuals to let other people know about their discoveries</u> easily and with less chance of getting into serious trouble.
Direct and well-supported judgement (Level 4)	The work of individuals like Vesalius was important in bringing about progress in anatomy <u>but it did not do much to improve treatments at the time because not all doctors believed it and anyway important discoveries like germ theory were still in the future.</u>

Comments

This answer ought to be worth at least 11 marks. Notice that it does not include all Renaissance individuals because the question doesn't ask for this. It only asks for examples. The answer shows an understanding that other factors were important but it only gives examples. The last paragraph goes back to the question and answers it directly with a judgement based on new knowledge. You could just as easily have based your judgement on the knowledge already used in paragraphs two and three.

There is always more than one way to produce a top-level answer in history

Key features in the development of medicine during the later Middle Ages and Renaissance

Cause

- Trained doctors treated mainly the wealthy but continued to believe in the **theory of the four humours.**
- **Paracelsus** believed that disease was caused by problems with chemicals in the body. Few people listened to him.
- The Christian Church taught that disease was **a punishment from God.**
- Astrology: a person's health was influenced by the **position of the stars and planets.**

Now in every man's body are four qualities: hot or cold, moist or dry. The amount of heat or cold is the cause of the colour of urine. Too much heat in the body makes the urine red. Moistness or dryness determine how thick or thin the urine is. If the patient's urine is, for example, red and thick it means that the blood is too hot and moist. If urine is red and thin this shows that choler is too hot and dry. If the urine appears white this is a sign of too much phlegm because phlegm is cold and moist. If the urine is white and thin it is a sign of too much melancholy for melancholy is cold and dry

Text from a fifteenth-century urine chart.

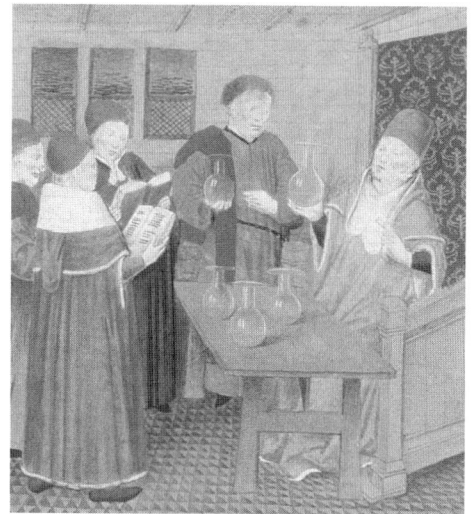

Cure

- **Paracelsus** experimented with chemical cures and believed that God created special plants to cure some diseases but few people listened to him.
- The Church said that **prayer** was the only cure and in extreme cases, such as the Black Death, flagellants whipped themselves to show God they were sorry.

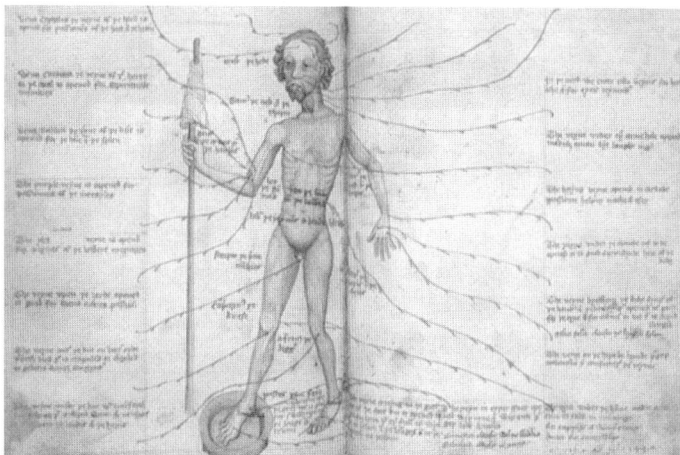

A chart showing all the places where doctors could cut the patient to draw blood

- **Vesalius** discovered many things about the human body but did not produce new cures for disease.
- The use of **herbs and plants** as purgatives or laxatives to restore the humours was also a common treatment, together with advice about diet and exercise.
- **Bleeding** a patient by cutting, cupping and using leeches was thought to keep the humours in balance.
- **Harvey** discovered the circulation of blood but did not produce new cures for disease.

Consider this question

How important was the Christian Church in hindering progress in the understanding of the causes and cures for diseases in the Middle Ages and Renaissance periods?
Support your answer with reasons and examples.

A mark scheme for assessing your answer might look like this:

Target: Assessing the importance of a factor in medicine

Level 1: Generalised answer (1–3 marks)

Level 2: Developed answer that explains the importance of the church *or* other factors (4–6 marks)

Level 3: Developed answer that explains the importance of the Church *and* other factors (7–9 marks)

Level 4: As Level 3 but with a direct judgement that is well-supported (10–12 marks)

Examiner's comments and level	A top-level answer might look like this:
Generalised (Level 1)	<u>The Christian Church hindered progress in understanding the causes and cures for disease because it said that Galen was always right.</u> The Church had great power. The Roman Empire had collapsed in about AD 300 and there was no strong government in Europe. This was the time of the Dark Ages when important medical knowledge from Hippocrates and Galen was lost in the West. This hindered progress. The Christian Church gradually took over. It taught that disease was a punishment from God, which could only be cured by prayer.
Developed points about the Church and other factors (Level 3)	The writings of Galen and Hippocrates were preserved in monasteries so natural ideas about observation and the four humours did survive but doctors could only use these ideas because the Church said they did not go against the Bible. The Church often punished people who used other ideas. Doctors would not listen to new ideas from people like Paracelsus because he burned Galen's books. Other ideas about the use of plants and astrology were also used but these did not help to cure patients because they were not correct.
Direct and well-supported judgement (Level 4)	The fall of the Roman Empire and wars during the Dark Ages also hindered the understanding of the causes and cures for disease because ancient ideas were lost. But it was the Christian Church that controlled Europe and hindered things the most.

Comment

Remember that there is never a single correct answer to a significant question like this. It is important to choose your examples and reasons carefully. In an alternative answer you might have said that the Church was very important in hindering progress early in the Middle Ages but by the time of the Renaissance it was losing its power. This allowed people like Vesalius and Paracelsus to make progress in understanding, even though they produced few, if any, effective cures.

Consider this question

How important was war in leading to progress in anatomy and surgery during the Renaissance period? Support your answer with reasons and examples.

A mark scheme for assessing your answer might look like this:

Target: Assessing the importance of a factor in surgery

Level 1: Generalised answer (1–3 marks)

Level 2: Developed answer that explains the importance of the war *or* other factors (4–6 marks)

Level 3: Developed answer that explains the importance of the war *and* other factors (7–9 marks)

Level 4: As Level 3 but with a direct judgement that is well supported (10–12 marks)

Examiner's comments and level	A top-level answer might look like this:
Generalised (Level 1)	There were many wars in Europe at this time. These gave surgeons the opportunity to try out new ideas and look at bodies on the battlefield. Normally it was difficult to dissect human bodies because the Church opposed this for religious reasons; but in war soldiers were injured and their wounds could be examined.
Developed answer on the importance of war (Level 2)	Ambroise Pare was an army surgeon who gained a lot of experience on the battlefield at this time. By accident he ran out of oil, which was normally used to prevent infection after amputation. He used an ointment that was less painful and more effective. He also used ligatures to tie up veins and prevent bleeding, which he found was better than a red hot iron.
Developed answer on the importance of other factors (Level 3)	At the end of the Middle Ages, during the Renaissance, the power of the Church began to decline and Andreas Vesalius was able to dissect bodies and show that Galen was wrong about some things, such as there being holes in the septum to allow blood to pass through the heart and about the human jaw bone. He published his ideas and this led to a much better understanding of anatomy.
Direct and well-supported judgement (Level 4)	So yes, war was very important in the development of surgery. So was chance in the case of Pare and the invention of printing so that books could spread new ideas quickly and widely but the decline of the power of the Church was much more important in allowing people like Vesalius to make progress in anatomy and question old ideas.

Revision Tip

Remember that the Middle Ages and Renaissance cover a long period of time. Look back at the revision tips on page 25. In the examination, the Renaissance will normally be treated as a separate period for questions. Make your own revision page on the Renaissance period.

How did medicine change and develop in the medieval and Renaissance world? What do you think?

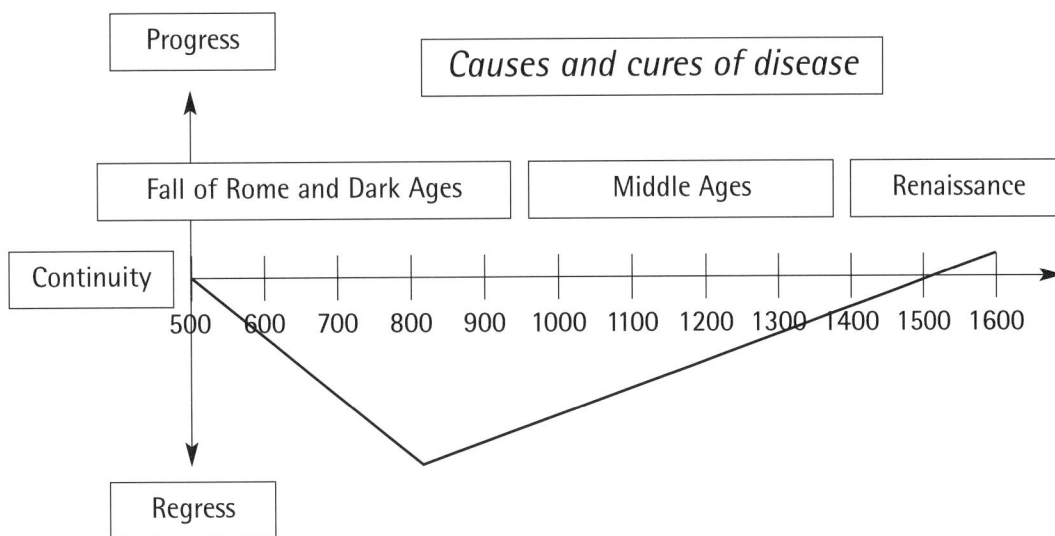

Progress

Causes and cures of disease

Fall of Rome and Dark Ages | Middle Ages | Renaissance

Continuity

500 600 700 800 900 1000 1100 1200 1300 1400 1500 1600

Regress

Comments

The chart above shows that ideas about the causes and cures of diseases regressed after the fall of Rome. The logical ideas of Hippocrates and Galen were lost for a while and medicine returned to the superstitious stage. This continued in the Middle Ages but the more logical ideas returned through monasteries and the Christian Church. After 1200, universities taught the ideas of Hippocrates and Galen to medical students. In the Renaissance, doctors like Paracelsus made a little progress.

Revision Tips

Some questions might ask you about how or why medicine developed more quickly or slowly during some periods rather than others. A chart like the one above might help you to see this more clearly.

Try drawing your own charts for:

- anatomy and surgery;
- public health in Britain.

Write important names and events on your charts at the appropriate dates.
Try extending your charts in to the ancient and prehistoric times.
Look back at page 24 of the chapter on the Ancient World and make some diagrams to show the factors that helped and hindered change in medieval and Renaissance times.

3. Medicine in the Industrial Revolution and the modern world

A summary of what you need to know about the Industrial Revolution and the modern world

Exam Paper	Sections A and B	Sections A and B	Section C
Time ╱ Theme	Cause, prevention and cure of disease	Practices of anatomy and surgery	Public health in Britain
AD 1700 The Industrial Revolution			
AD 1800	Jenner – vaccination		Growth of towns and industry
Crimean War	Pasteur – germ theory Koch – Bacteriology	Simpson – chloroform Nightingale – nursing Lister – antiseptic surgery	Cholera epidemics 1848 Public Health Act Edwin Chadwich John Snow Octavia Hill 1875 Public Health Act
AD 1900	Ehrlich – magic bullets	Halstead Aseptic surgery	Booth and Rowntree Lloyd-George Liberal Social Reforms
First World War	Fleming – penicillin Florey and Chain		
Second World War	Wilkins, Watson and Crick – DNA AIDS epidemic	McIndoe – plastic surgery Barnard – heart transplant	Beveridge and Bevan National Health Service
AD 2000			

✎ Revision Tips

The Industrial Revolution and the modern world cover only a short period of time compared with the ancient world and the medieval and Renaissance periods. They will usually be the last periods in the history of medicine that you study. Beware. These periods contain a lot of detail. They include the work of a great many key individuals and most of the material on Section C: Public Health in Britain. You can divide them into three sections:

- The Enlightenment (1700–1800) – a growing belief that science and reason would lead to progress.
- Industrialisation (1800–1900) – germ theory was discovered and government action on public health in Britain began.
- The twentieth century (1900–2000) – the use of science and technology in medicine accelerated and government concerns about issues like AIDS and genetic engineering became world wide.

Key features of society in the Industrial Revolution and the modern world

The growth of towns, industry and population

▼ SOURCE A

Manchester in 1850

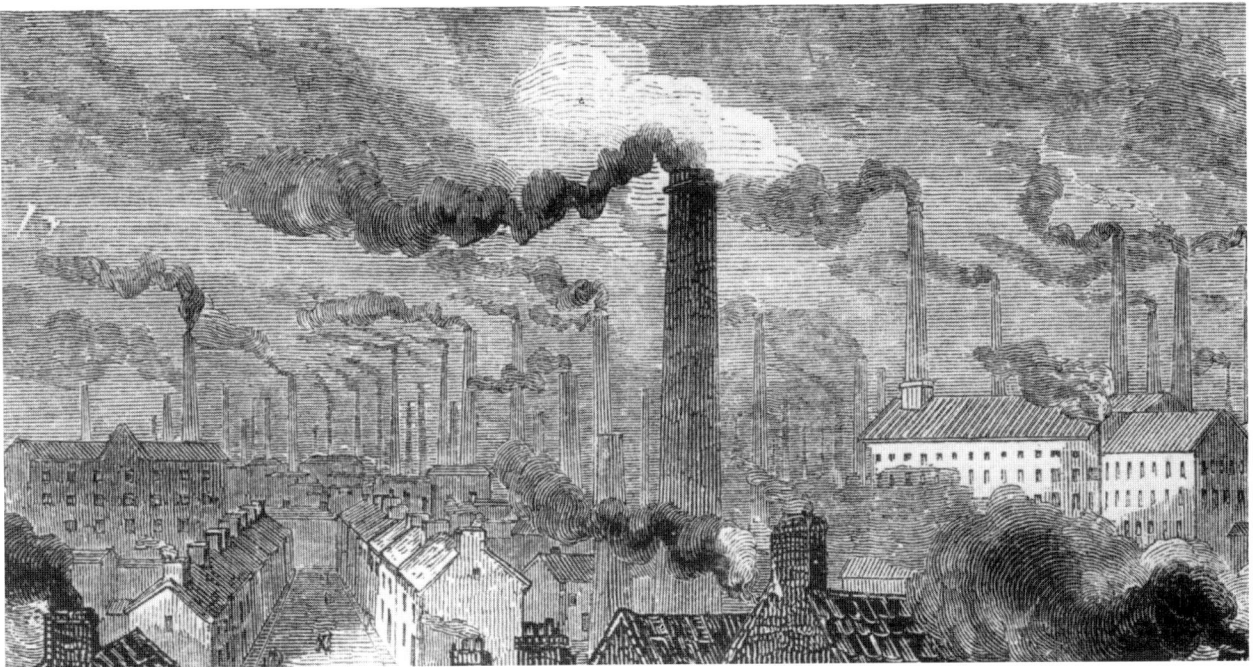

The development of science and technology

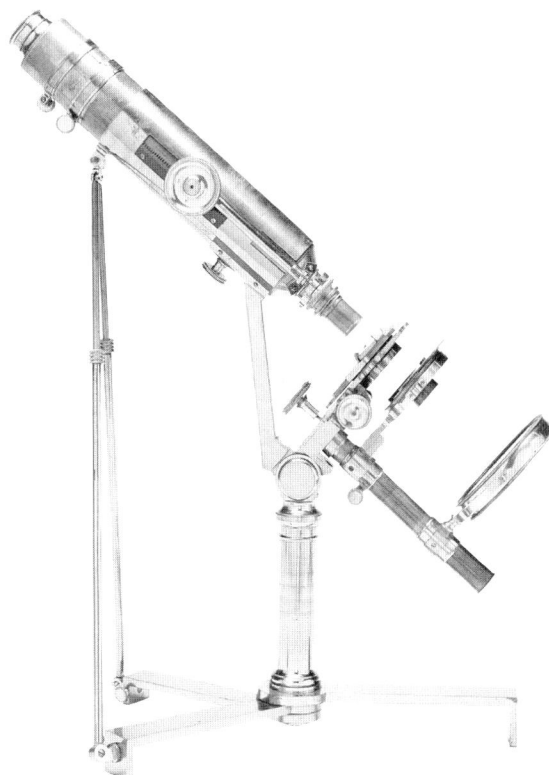

▶ SOURCE B

A microscope produced in 1826

45

The impact of war

▼ SOURCE C

Flames encircle a Vickers Wellington Bomber during the Second World War

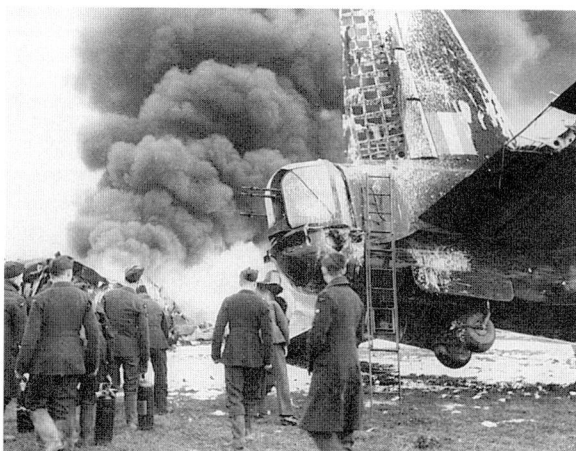

Government action

▼ SOURCE D

A poster produced by the Liberal government seeking support for their policy of compulsory National Insurance in 1911

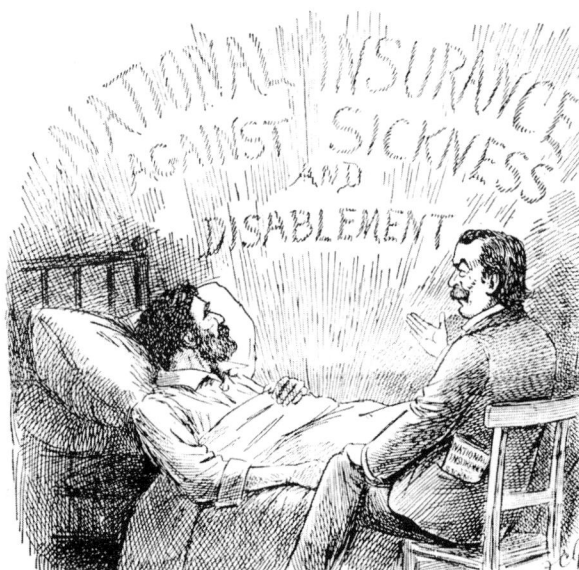

✎ Revision Tips

Each of these sources shows a reason or factor leading to developments in medicine during the period 1700–2000.

Use each factor as a heading. Underneath each heading list as many events and individuals connected with that factor and the development of medicine as you can.

Section C of the examination paper will set you questions on public health in Britain.

Consider this question, which might be the first part of a public health question.

What can you learn from Source A about the problems of public health in towns and cities in the early nineteenth century? Explain your answer using Source A and your own knowledge.

A mark scheme for assessing your answer might look like this:

Target: Comprehension and inference from an historical source

Level 1: Answer that selects detail from the source (1 mark)

Level 2: Answer that draws a simple inference from the source (2–3 marks)

Level 3: Answer that sets the source in the context of knowledge (4–5 marks)

Examiner's comments and level	A top-level answer might look like this:
Selects detail (Level 1)	<u>The city looks very crowded and smoky.</u>
Simple inference (Level 2)	Public health was a problem because <u>nobody has done anything about the smoke and with people being crowded together in these conditions</u> diseases would spread quickly.
Sets source in the context of knowledge (Level 3)	The source shows that the government was not taking any action to improve public health. The <u>factories were dangerous places with unfenced machinery which led to many injuries and dust in the air leading to lung diseases. The housing for the workers was near to the factories. Many families shared a house. Most houses had no running water or toilets. The 1848 Public Health Act was not compulsory and made little difference in most towns.</u> Sewage would be in the street and would run into the water supplies causing more problems.

Consider this question, which might be the second part of a public health question

Between 1831 and 1850, cholera killed almost 100,000 people in Britain.

Explain two reasons why cholera killed so many people in the early nineteenth century.

There are many reasons or factors which could explain why cholera had such a great effect at this time. You only need to explain two in some detail to get full marks for your answer. Find some information on each of these reasons:

- the government's policy of *laissez-faire*;
- the lack of understanding about what really caused diseases like cholera;
- treatments based on theories about poisonous air or religion;
- the effects of crowded conditions, poor sanitation and lack of clean water supplies;
- the growth of trade and industry.

For each developed explanation you would get 4 marks.
E.g. People did not know the real cause because Pasteur did not discover germ theory until after 1850 so they had many ideas on what to do about cholera but none of them worked.
Now try writing your own answer using two of the other reasons.

Consider this question which might be the final part of a public health question

Had public health in towns and cities improved by 1900? Explain your answer.

A mark scheme for assessing your answer might look like this:

Target: Understanding the idea of progress

Level 1: Generalised answer (1–3 marks)

Level 2: *Either*
       Developed answer that agrees or disagrees
       Or
       Simple answer that agrees and disagrees (4–6 marks)

Level 3: Developed answer that agrees and disagrees (7–9 marks)

Level 4: As Level 3 but with a direct and well-supported judgement (10–12 marks)

Examiner's comments and level	A top-level answer might look like this:
Generalised answer (Level 1)	<u>Yes, the government had begun to take action to clean up towns and cities</u> after 1850.
Developed answer that agrees (Level 2)	Edwin Chadwick had led the Board of Health from 1848. It tried to improve water supply and sewerage in many large towns but it did not have the power to make changes compulsory. Many councils did not want to increase rates to pay for facilities for the <u>poor, so public health did not improve.</u>
Developed answer that agrees (Level 3)	In the 1850s several things happened which led to improvements. Dr Snow linked cholera with dirty water, Pasteur proved that germs caused disease and Sir John Simon became the first government medical officer. On top of this, working men got the vote in the 1860s <u>so then public health began to improve fast.</u>
Direct and well-supported judgement (Level 4)	In 1875 the Public Health Act made it compulsory for councils to provide water sewage and drainage. There were also laws so that councils could knock down slums and set up public parks. <u>Public health had improved by 1900 because of all these things and because there were now health and medical inspectors to enforce the rules.</u>

Revision Tips

When revising for questions on public health in the nineteenth century make sure you are clear about the main facts:

- cholera outbreaks;
- the work of Edwin Chadwick, Dr Snow and Sir John Simon;
- details of the Public Health Acts of 1848 and 1875;
- developments in the understanding of the causes of disease.

Key developments in the prevention of disease in the eighteenth and nineteenth centuries

Revision Tips

This is the specified topic for Section A in 2003 and a strong possibility for questions on Section B in other years. Look back at pages 3, 4, 5 and 6 of the Introduction and review the Section A question and mark scheme on opposition to Jenner's discovery of smallpox vaccination.

Now study the sources and information below which develop this topic.

Louis Pasteur (1822–1895)

- Professor of Chemistry in France.
- Used microscope to show local wine growers that wine went off because of micro-organisms (germs).
- 1861 – published his experiments, which showed that germs were present in the air all the time and were the cause of decay not the result of it.
- 1865 – Lister used this idea to help prevent infection in surgery by soaking dressings and instruments and spraying the air with carbolic acid.
- 1880s – produced vaccines for chicken cholera, anthrax and rabies.

▶ **SOURCE E**

Pasteur after his experiments with the swan-necked flask said

There is now no circumstances known in which it can be proved that microsopic beings came into the world without germs.

Robert Koch (1843–1910)

- German doctor interested in research into germs.
- Used a microscope and found a way of staining and growing germs so that they could be photographed through it.
- 1882 – identified the germ causing tuberculosis.
- 1884 – identified the germ causing cholera.
- 1885 – an international conference refused to examine Koch's findings.
- Koch's methods were used by other researchers to identify the germs that cause many killer diseases.

▶ **SOURCE F**

A cartoon from 1880 showing Robert Koch beating infectious disease

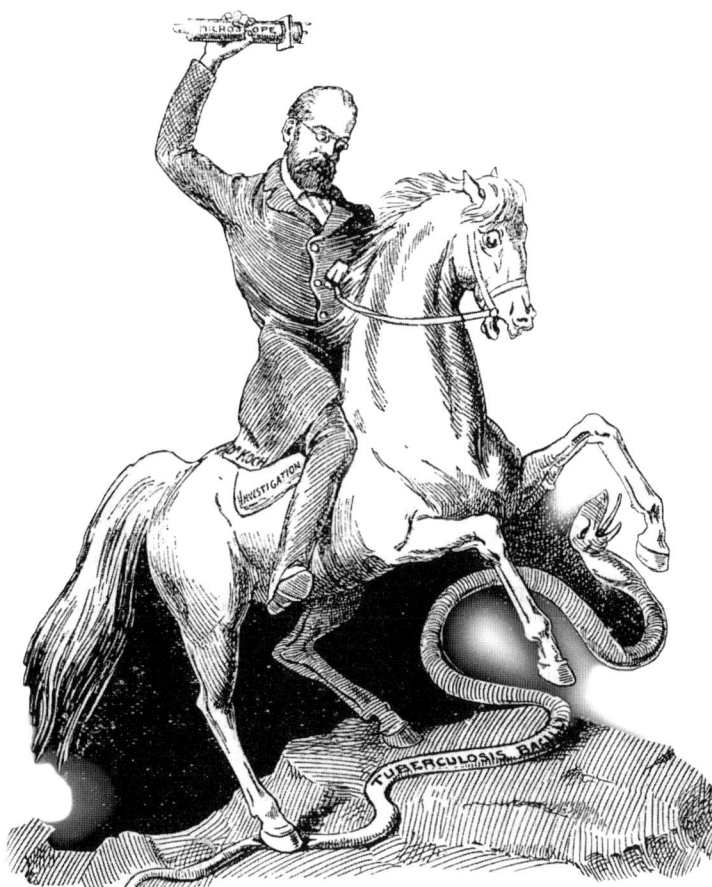

How important was the role of individuals in the prevention of disease?

- Jenner, Pasteur and Koch were very important in the fight against disease in the eighteenth and nineteenth centuries but their discoveries did not lead to immediate cures for diseases like cholera, tuberculosis, pneumonia and diptheria.
- Government action in the nineteenth century played a big part in helping to prevent disease (see pages 47 and 48 in this chapter).
- Developments in science and technology, such as improvements in microscopes and the chemical industry, were also important.

- The Crimean War (1853–1856) helped Florence Nightingale to improve hospitals so that patients were less likely to die of a disease they caught in hospital.
- The Franco–Prussian War (1870–1871) produced competition between France and Germany, which in turn produced rivalry between Pasteur and Koch, which may have spurred them on.

Remember that developments in medicine are complicated. Always consider the different factors and how they worked together.

Consider this question, which might be one of the parts of the question in Section A.

Source A on page 3 of the Introduction suggests that people did not accept Jenner's ideas on smallpox vaccination because they did not understand them. **Source F on page 49 of this chapter** shows Robert Koch as a champion of medicine in using science to battle against infectious diseases. Does **Source F** show that people no longer believed the ideas shown in **Source A**?

Explain your answer using the **two sources and your own knowledge**.

A mark scheme for assessing your answer might look like this:

Target: Explaining differences between sources

Level 1: Answer that describes the content (1–2 marks)

Level 2: Answer that makes a simple inference from the source(s) (3–5 marks)

Level 3: Answer that makes a detailed and complex inference (6–7 marks)

Level 4: Answer that sets the sources in the context of knowledge (8–9 marks)

Examiner's comments and level	A top-level answer might look like this:
Describes content (Level 1)	<u>Source A shows cows growing out of people's bodies after they have been vaccinated for smallpox and</u> Source F shows Koch attacking tuberculosis with his microscope.
Makes inference from source (Level 2)	<u>Source F shows that people believed that doctors were doing good work because Koch is shown as a champion over disease but in Source</u> A people did not understand what Jenner was doing and thought it was stupid.
Complex inference-based on source type (Level 3)	Both the sources are cartoons. Source A shows that people believed medicine was a bad thing and Source F shows that people believed medicine was a good thing. <u>But they are only the views of the cartoonists. They may, however, speak for many people.</u> But they do not tell us what most people really believed.

Uses knowledge to put sources in context (Level 4)	<u>At the time of Source A, Pasteur had not discovered the germ theory</u> and Jenner could not really explain how his vaccination worked, but by the time of Source F germ theory was discovered so it is probably true that most people no longer believed the ideas shown in Source A. New ideas do take time to be accepted, however, so we cannot be 100% certain that some people did not still believe ideas like those in Source A.

Comments

Remember that answers do not have to cover every level to gain the top level. In this particular answer only the second or the third and last paragraphs would be needed. This is all the question asks for.

Consider this question, which might be the final interpretation part of the question in Section A

Pasteur's discovery of germ theory was the most important factor in the development of the prevention of diseases in the nineteenth century.

Use Source B (page 45), Sources E and F (page 49) and your own knowledge to explain why you agree or disagree with this interpretation?

A mark scheme for assessing your answer might look like this:

Target: Evaluating an interpretation of the past

Level 1: *Either*

Answer that extracts information from the sources to agree or disagree
Or
Answer that makes general statements using knowledge (1–3 marks)

Level 2: *Either*

Simple answer that extracts information from sources *and* uses knowledge
Or
Answer that develops one or more points using sources *or* knowledge (4–8 marks)

Level 3: Answer that develops one or more points using sources *and* knowledge (9–12 marks)

Level 4: Developed answer that assesses the interpretation using sources *and* knowledge to reach a balanced judgement (13–15 marks)

Examiner's comments and level	A top-level answer might look like this:
General statement using knowledge (Level 1)	This interpretation is true because Pasteur's discovery <u>found the true cause of disease and disproved spontaneous generation.</u>
Developed points using knowledge (Level 2)	People were against <u>Jenner's ideas because he could not show exactly how they worked.</u> Pasteur solved this problem with his swan-necked flask experiments. He proved that germs were in the air all the time and that they were the cause of disease and infection not the result. <u>He then went on to find vaccines for chicken cholera, anthrax and rabies. His ideas were used by Lister. He used carbolic acid</u> to kill germs so that patients did not get infections after surgery. So I agree that germ theory and its discovery were very important.
Developed points using sources (Level 3)	Source B shows a microscope. <u>Pasteur would not have been able to make his discovery if this had not been invented and improved. Also Source F shows a cartoon of Koch as the champion over disease.</u> It was his methods that led to the discovery of the germs causing TB and cholera. Other people were then able to find ways of killing them.
Balanced judgement based on sources and knowledge (Level 4)	I agree with the interpretation because <u>the microscope had been around for a while but germ theory was not yet discovered. Source F is a cartoon that probably tries to exaggerate Koch's importance. It was Pasteur's proof shown in Source E that was the most important factor.</u>

Key developments in medicine from 1700 to 2000

Use of speed and skill

▶ **SOURCE A**

An operation in 1793 before anaesthetics

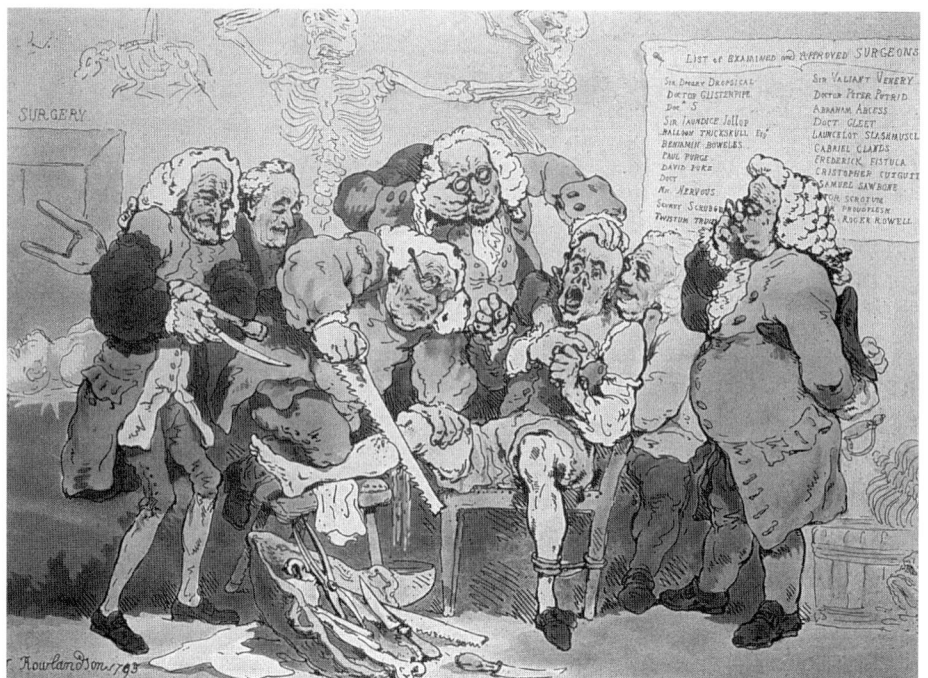

✎ Revision Tips

Early operations were limited by three major problems:

- Pain meant that patients had to be restrained because they suffered and struggled throughout the operation and surgeons had to work quickly.
- Blood loss lead to shock, which often killed the patient.
- Infection often got into the open wounds and killed the patient, even if they did not suffer severe blood loss.

Surgery was the last resort.

✎ Revision Tips

Anaesthetics were first used widely by surgeons in the 1850s. Some people opposed their use because:

- ether irritated the lungs and gave off inflammable gas;
- chloroform gave patients headaches;
- many people died from being given too much;
- some believed that God meant childbirth to be painful;
- at first patients still died from blood loss, infection or operations that were too risky.

Use of anaesthetics

▶ **SOURCE B**

From a letter written to James Simpson in 1853 by one of Queen Victoria's doctors

The queen had chloroform exhibited to her during her last confinement. It acted admirably. Her Majesty was greatly pleased with the effect and she has certainly had a better recovery. I know this information will please you and I have little doubt that it will lead to a more general use of chloroform in the midwifery practice.

Use of antiseptics

▼ **SOURCE C**

A drawing of a carbolic spray such as the one used in operations by Joseph Lister

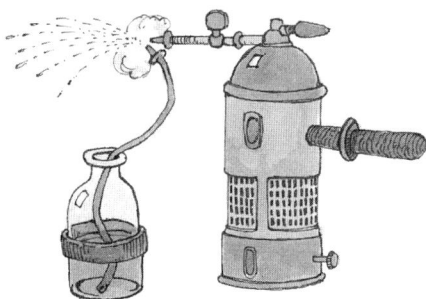

✎ Revision Tips

Lister first used carbolic acid in 1867. His approach improved the recovery rate of patients after surgery because fewer suffered from infections. Not all surgeons used his methods because being sprayed with carbolic was unpleasant and damaged the hands.

Robert Koch recommended cleaning the tools and operating theatre of all germs before an operation. This became known as aseptic surgery. The same approach was also developed by an American surgeon called Halstead after 1889.

Improvements in hospitals and medical care

▶ **SOURCE D**

A nurse caring for a newly born baby in a modern hospital maternity ward

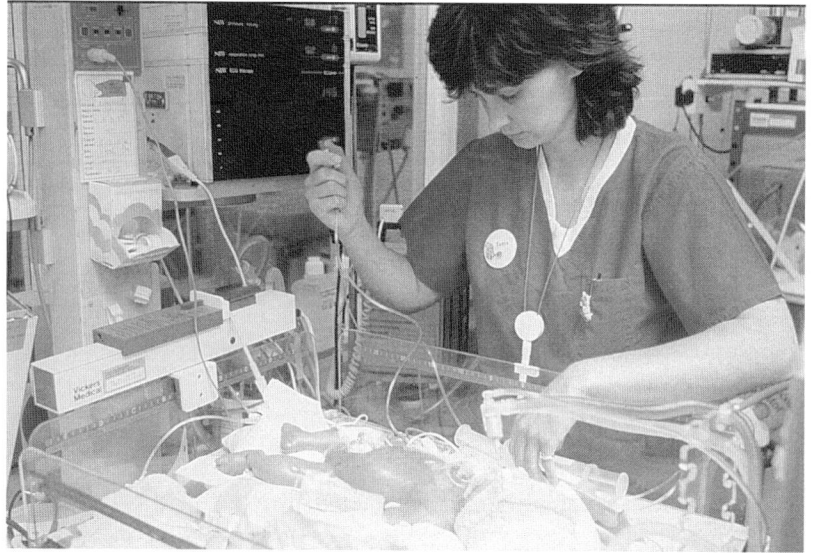

Revision Tips

- In the eighteenth century, some rich people believed it was their duty to use their money to help poor sick people, so they paid for hospitals to be built.
- In the middle of the nineteenth century, Chadwick convinced many people that if the poor were kept healthy they would save the country money because they would work harder and want fewer benefits.

- Florence Nightingale, who lived from 1820 to 1910, showed that training nurses and cleaning up hospitals would reduce the death rate. In 1860 she started the first training school for nurses.
- 1948 — introduction of the National Health Service in Britain, offering free treatment and services to all.

World health issues

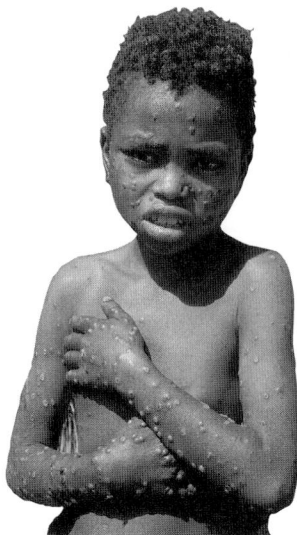

Revision Tips

- In 1948, 61 member countries of the United Nations signed the constitution of the World Health Organisation (WHO), agreeing to help all peoples to reach the highest possible level of health.
- Between 1967 and 1980 smallpox was eradicated across the world.
- WHO now campaigns against other diseases that are a worldwide threat, such as HIV and AIDS.

▲ **SOURCE E**

A smallpox sufferer in Africa sometime in the twentieth century before the disease was eradicated

Genetic therapy and engineering

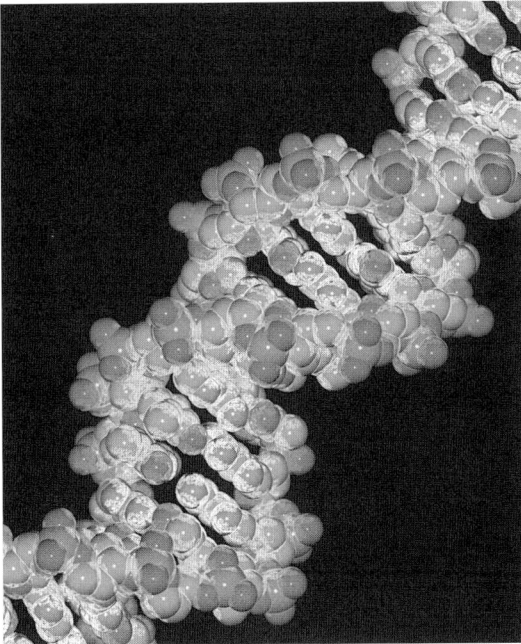

▲ SOURCE F
The double helix structure of DNA

Consider this question

Does Source E show that the work of Edward Jenner on vaccination was a failure?
Explain your answer **using Source E and your own knowledge.**

A mark scheme for assessing your answer can be found on page 50.

Consider this question

What does Source A show you about the problems of surgery before 1793?

Look back at the mark scheme on page 46 and try writing a top-level answer to this question.

Consider this question

Why did surgery improve in the nineteenth century?

A mark scheme for assessing your answer might look like this:

Target: Understanding the reasons for change in medicine

Level 1: Generalised answer (1–3 marks)

Level 2: *Either*
　　　　Answer that describes the changes
　　　　Or
　　　　Answer that explains one reason in detail
　　　　Or
　　　　Answer that lists several different reasons (4–6 marks)

Level 3: Answer that explains several different reasons (7–9 marks)

Level 4: Answer that links several explanations together to make a supported judgement (10–12 marks)

Examiner's comments and level	A top-level answer might look like this:
Generalised answer (Level 1)	Before surgery could improve, surgeons had to overcome three main problems. These were: pain, infection and blood loss.
Explains one reason in detail (Level 2)	The nineteenth century was the period of the industrial revolution when many important discoveries were made, which helped doctors to solve the above problems. The chemical industry led to the discovery of gases like nitrous oxide then later ether and chloroform. Anaesthetics became popular with some surgeons when it was used by Queen Victoria in 1853 during childbirth.
	Anaesthetics did not lead to immediate improvements in surgery, however, because patients still died from infection and the anaesthetics sometimes had adverse side-effects.
Explains several different reasons (Level 3) *Supported judgement (Level 4)*	It was not until the 1860s that the real turning point came when Lister heard about germ theory from Pasteur. It had also been noticed that the smell of infection in wounds was like sewage, which was treated with carbolic acid. He used carbolic acid in a spray during operations and to soak bandages and found that fewer patients died from infection. Later, Koch and Halstead recommended aseptic surgery and this brought great improvements. <u>The final problem of blood loss was not solved until the twentieth century, however, the discovery of germ theory and its link to infection was a turning point for surgery at the time.</u>

Top marks in the level are for supporting the answer with detailed and accurate knowledge.

The impact of science and technology in medicine since 1900

This is the specified aspect of Medicine through Time for Section A of the 2005 examination paper.

The impact of the First World War on medical technology

▶ SOURCE A

A Petite Curie

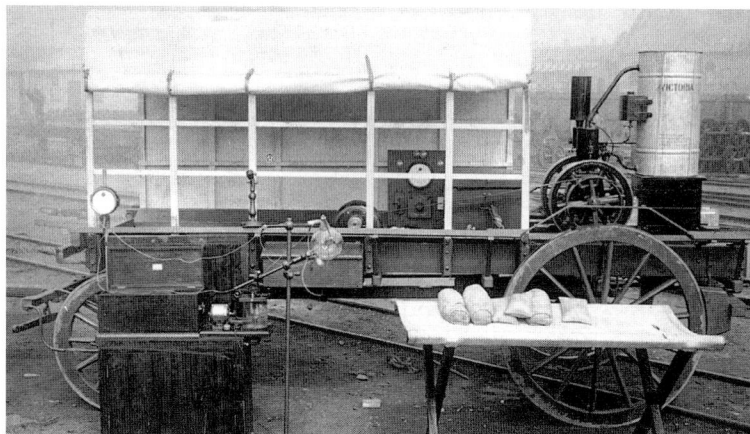

The application of science to medicine

- 1895 – Rontgen uses X-rays.
- 1903 – Electrocardiograph or heart monitor invented.
- 1908 – First successful blood transfusion using the blood groups discovered by Landsteiner in 1901.
- 1931 – Electron microscope invented.
- 1937 – First blood bank set up in Chicago.
- 1967 – Dr Barnard completed the first successful human heart transplant.

Medical research and chance:

- 1908 – Ehrlich's research team discovers Salvarsan 606. The first magic bullet.
- 1929 – Fleming accidentally discovers the properties of penicillin.
- 1935 – Domagk successfully tested Prontosil on his daughter. The second magic bullet.
- 1941 – Florey and Chain tried penicillin on a policeman. They proved that it worked to combat blood poisoning but ran out of the substance before they could save the policeman's life.
- During the Second World War, Andrew Moyer, with United States government support, discovered a process for the industrial production of penicillin, which saved thousands of soldiers' lives.

The roles of individuals and chance in the development of medical science

▶ **SOURCE B**

The world's first penicillin factory in the Sir William Dunn School of Pathology, Oxford University

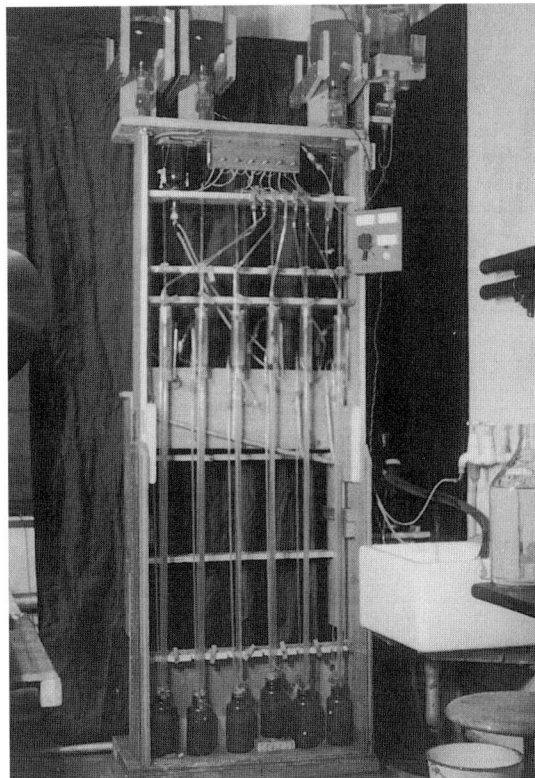

Alternatives to scientific medicine

▶ SOURCE C

The Prince of Wales speaking to a patient with breast cancer who is receiving aromatherapy treatment at the Haven Trust's support centre in London

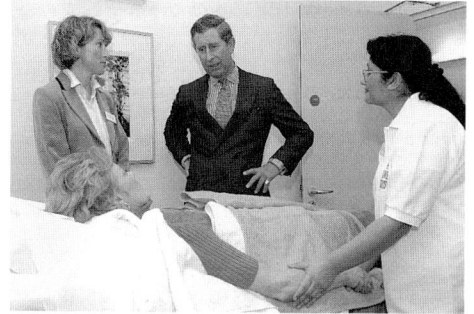

Alternatives to modern scientific medical treatment

An increasing number of people have rejected medicine based on modern science and technology, preferring to use older or alternative treatments based on acupuncture or herbs and plants. The reasons for this are complicated. Some of them are:

- the adverse side-effects of some modern drugs;
- the failure of some modern treatments to stop some cancers and diseases;
- the dangers and risks of modern surgery;
- long waiting lists for treatments through the NHS.

Consider these questions

What can you learn from Source A about the use of science in medicine at the beginning of the twentieth century?

- Use the mark scheme on pages 5 and 6 of the Introduction to write a top-level answer to this question.
- Remember that the question does not ask for knowledge so you must make a complex inference to reach the top level.

How does Source F on page 55 show that the use of science in medicine had developed since the beginning of the twentieth century?
Explain your answer **using the sources and your own knowledge.**

- Use the mark scheme on page 28 of The Medieval and Renaissance World to write a top-level answer to this question.
- This question does require knowledge as well as the sources to reach the top level.
- You could mention the developments in the use of X-rays and microscopes in particular.
- Don't forget the limitations of the sources.

Sources A and F suggest that science has led to progress in medicine since 1900.
Source C shows that people in the late 1900s have turned to alternative treatments.
Does Source C mean that science has failed?
Explain your answer **using the sources and your own knowledge.**

- Use the mark scheme on page 50 of this section to write a top-level answer to this question.
- This question does require knowledge as well as the sources to reach the top level.
- You could mention the problems of using scientific treatments such as the cost and possible side-effects.

Consider this question

Scientific research and discovery has been the most important factor in the development of medicine since 1900.

Use the **sources on pages 56, 57 and 58 and your own knowledge** to explain why you agree or disagree with this interpretation.

A mark scheme for assessing your answer might look like this:

Target: Evaluating an interpretation of the past

Level 1: *Either*

A basic answer that extracts information from sources to agree or disagree

Or

Answer that makes general or undeveloped statements from knowledge (1–3 marks)

Level 2: *Either*

A simple answer that extracts information from sources *and* own knowledge

Or

Answer that develops one or more points using sources *or* knowledge (4–8 marks)

Level 3: Answer that develops one or more points using sources *and* own knowledge (9–12 marks)

Level 4: Developed answer that assesses the interpretation using sources and knowledge to reach a balanced judgement (13–15 marks)

Examiner's comments and level	A top-level answer might look like this:
Undeveloped using sources or own knowledge (Level 2)	I think this statement is partly true because scientists like Ehrlich and Fleming have done a lot of research, which has led to the discovery of drugs like Salvarsan 606 and penicillin, which can kill nearly all infections and diseases and have saved millions of lives.
Develops several points using sources and knowledge (Level 3)	Source A shows that individuals and war have also been important factors in developing medicine. In the First World War, Marie Curie gave up her research on radium to set up mobile X-ray stations on the battlefield. This helped to develop the use of X-rays in medicine and surgery which might not have happened so quickly without the war.
	In the Second World War it was injuries to fighter pilots that led McIndoe to develop plastic surgery at the East Grinstead Hospital. But war also slowed down work on radium treatment.
Assesses interpretation to reach a balanced judgement (Level 4)	Source C shows that scientific discoveries cannot cure all diseases like cancer, but overall most people turn to modern drugs and surgery for cures, and discoveries like DNA are leading to new scientific breakthroughs all the time. Science has been the most important factor in development.

The roles of individuals in developments in public health in Britain during the twentieth century

Failure of government action in the nineteenth century

Charles Booth and Seebohm Rowntree:

- Both were rich businessmen who did social research into poverty in Britain at the beginning of the twentieth century.
- Both argued that the government should take action to improve the health of working people.
- Both men encouraged David Lloyd-George and the Liberal Party to take action:
  - 1908, Old Age Pensions Act.
  - 1911, National Health Insurance Act.

The impact of war

William Beveridge:

- Worked for the government to organise unemployment insurance after the 1911 Act.
- Produced the Beveridge Report in 1942.
- Argued for full health insurance for everyone.

Successful government action

Aneurin Bevan:

- Son of a Welsh coal miner.
- Minister of Health for the Labour Government elected after the Second World War.
- Introduced the Bill that created the National Health Service in 1946.
- National Health Service began in 1948 with free treatment and services for all including:
  - hospitals
  - eye tests and spectacles
  - dental treatment
  - visits to local doctors
  - medicine on prescription
  - maternity and child welfare
  - ambulance emergency services.

▼ **SOURCE A**

From Seebohm Rowntree, Poverty: A Study of Town Life, *1901*

> In this land of great wealth, during a time of growing prosperity, probably more than a quarter of the population are living in poverty.

▼ **SOURCE B**

From the front page of the Daily Mirror, *2 December 1942*

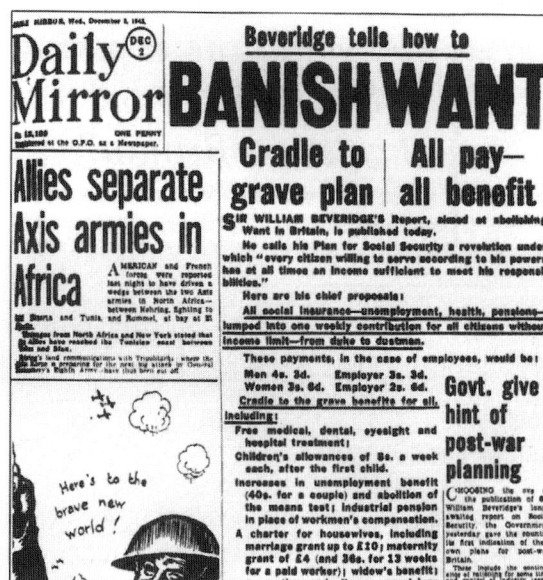

▼ **SOURCE C**

Aneurin Bevan on the introduction of the bill for a National Health Service in 1946

> Medical treatment should be made available to rich and poor alike in accordance with medical need and no other criteria. Worry about money in time of sickness is a serious hindrance to recovery, apart from its unnecessary cruelty.

Consider these questions

Explain two reasons why governments took action to improve public health in Britain during the early twentieth century.

A mark scheme for assessing your answer might look like this:

Target: Understanding causation

Level 1: Generalised answer (1 mark)

Level 2: Basic answer (2–3 marks)

Level 3: Developed answer (4 marks)

Examiner's comments and level	A top-level answer might look like this:
Generalised answer (Level 2)	Governments took action because reports by people like Booth and Rowntree showed politicians that many people were living in poverty.
Basic answer (Level 2)	They argued that poverty was caused by low wages and unemployment, which was often linked with ill health and bad living conditions.
Second cause developed (Level 3 x 2)	By the early twentieth century, many people could vote and politicians knew they would not get elected if they did not provide better public health. They also had problems getting enough fit men to fight in the Boer and First World Wars so they knew they had to take action to defend the country.

If you are asked for two reasons you will be awarded up to 4 marks for each one you explain.

What can you learn from Source B about the importance of war in the setting up of the National Health Service in 1948? Explain your answer using Source B and your own knowledge.

- Look at the example answer on page 34 of The Medieval and Renaissance World then try to write a top-level answer to this question.
- Remember that the question asks for knowledge as well as use of the source.
- You might want to mention the soldier shown in the source and the Beveridge Report.
- Show your knowledge of the effects of the Second World War.

Why was the setting up of the National Health Service in 1948 a turning point in dealing with public health in Britain?

- Questions about turning points need to be answered by making comparisons between what public health was like before the NHS and what it was like after the NHS had been set up. Only then can you explain why the NHS was a turning point.

Reviewing your study of medicine through time

✎ Final Revision Tips

Look back at pages 6 and 7 of the Introduction and consider what sort of questions you might be asked in the examination.

Think about them in groups like this:

- **Knowledge** – what changed and what stayed the same or got worse (keep going over the lists at the beginning of each section and adding details to your own lists)?
- **Understanding factors** – why did things change or stay the same (look back at page 24 of The Ancient World and make sure you have drawn your own diagrams for each of the sections of the book)?
- **Understanding time** – when did things change quickly, slowly or not at all (look back at page 43 of The Medieval and Renaissance World and make sure you have drawn charts with explanations for each section of the book)?
- **Understanding evidence** – what do different sources tell you about change or the lack of it (look back at page 31 of The Medieval and Renaissance World and some of the source questions you have answered)?
- **Understanding interpretations** – why do historians disagree about what happened and which opinion is more likely to be correct (look back at page 31 of The Medieval and Renaissance World and look again at some of the example questions on interpretations)?

How has medicine developed from prehistoric times to the present day?

Finally you need to get an overview of the whole study.

It is easy to see the development of medicine as a steady line of progress from prehistoric to modern times. It is important to study the details in the previous pages of this revision book to find examples of:

- Regression (times of war such as after the fall of the Roman Empire).
- Stagnation (the Middle Ages when the Church controlled ideas).
- Continuity (the use of plants and herbs, which is still popular in some places today).

Remember that the development of medicine is complicated and open to interpretation. Examiners will expect top-level answers to show this.

Now look back over some of the sample questions and answers before your examination.

Section A Specified Aspects of Medicine through Time

2003: Developments in the prevention of disease in the eighteenth and nineteenth centuries

Source A on page 3 of the Introduction suggests that people did not accept Jenner's ideas on smallpox vaccination because they did not understand them. **Source F on page 49 of this section** shows Robert Koch as a champion of medicine in using science to battle against infectious diseases. Does **Source F** show that people no longer believed the ideas shown in **Source A**?
Explain your answer using the **two sources and your own knowledge**. (*Modern World, page 50*)

'Pasteur's discovery of germ theory was the most important factor in the development of the prevention of diseases in the nineteenth century.'
Use **Source B (page 45), Sources E and F (page 49) and your own knowledge** to explain why you agree or disagree with this interpretation? (*Modern World, page 51*)

Does **Source E** show that the work of Edward Jenner on vaccination was a failure? (*Modern World, page 55*)

2004: The impact of religion on medicine in the Middle Ages

How does Source C show that Islamic religion had a different impact on medical ideas from Christian religion in the early Middle Ages? **Explain your answer using Sources B and C and your own knowledge.** (*Medieval and Renaissance, page 27*)

Read the following extract adapted from *Medicine through Time*, a school textbook written by Joe Scott in 1990, and then answer the question that follows.

> *The Christian Church taught that it was part of people's religious duty to care for the sick but until 1200 it did little to help in the study of medicine.*

Study Sources D, E, F and G. **Use the sources and your own knowledge** to explain why you agree or disagree with this interpretation. (*Medieval and Renaissance, page 30*)

2005: The impact of science and technology in medicine since 1900

What can you learn from Source A about the use of science in medicine at the beginning of the twentieth century? (*Modern World, page 58*)

How does Source F on page 55 show that the use of science in the development of surgery in medicine had developed since the beginning of the twentieth century? (*Modern World, page 58*)

Sources A and F suggest that science has led to steady progress in surgery since 1900.
Source C shows that people in the late 1900s have turned to alternative treatments.
Does Source C mean that science had failed?
Explain your answer **using the sources and your own knowledge.** (*Modern World, page 58*)

Section B Medicine through Time: changing ideas and practices in the cause, prevention and cure of disease and infection, with changes in the understanding and practices of anatomy and surgery

How does each of the sources help you to understand medicine in prehistoric times? (*Ancient World, page 10*)

Does Source D show that ideas about medicine had changed between prehistoric times and the Ancient Egyptian period? Explain your answer **using Sources B and D and your own knowledge.** (*Ancient World, page 12*)

What does Source D tell you about the cures used by the Ancient Egyptians? (*Ancient World, page 21*)

How important was the work of Hippocrates in explaining the cause and cure of disease in the ancient world? (*Ancient World, page 22*)

Why did the Romans believe in preventing rather than curing disease? (*Ancient World, page 23*)

How does Source B help you to understand medicine in the early Middle Ages? (*Medieval and Renaissance, page 26*)

How important was the work of Renaissance individuals in bringing about progress in medicine by 1700? Support your answer with reasons and examples. (*Medieval and Renaissance, page 39*)

How important was the Christian Church in hindering progress in the understanding of the causes and cures for diseases in the Middle Ages and Renaissance periods?
Support your answer with reasons and examples. (*Medieval and Renaissance, page 41*)

How important was war in leading to progress in anatomy and surgery during the Renaissance period? Support your answer with reasons and examples. (*Medieval and Renaissance, page 42*)

What does Source A show you about the problems of surgery before 1793? (*Modern World, page 55*)

Why did surgery improve in the nineteenth century? (*Modern World, page 55*)

Section C Public Health in Britain

What can you learn from Sources C and D about public health in Roman Britain? Explain your answer **using the sources and your own knowledge.** (*Ancient World, page 17*)

What can you learn from Source A about government action on public health in towns and cities in the Middle Ages? Explain your answer **using Source A and your own knowledge.** (*Medieval and Renaissance, page 33*)

Did public health in Britain generally get worse during the Middle Ages?
Explain your answer. (*Medieval and Renaissance, page 34*)

What can you learn from Source A about the problems of public health in towns and cities in the early nineteenth century? Explain your answer **using Source A and your own knowledge.** (*Modern World, page 46*)

Had public health in towns and cities improved by 1900? Explain your answer (*Modern World, page 47*)

Explain two reasons why governments took action to improve public health in Britain during the early twentieth century. (*Modern World, page 61*)

What can you learn from Source B about the importance of war in the setting up of the National Health Service in 1948? Explain your answer **using Source B and your own knowledge.** (*Modern World, page 61*)

Why was the setting up of the National Health Service in 1948 a turning point in dealing with public health in Britain? (*Modern World, page 61*)

Please note that the questions and mark schemes in this revision book have not been subjected to an AQA question paper evaluation committee. They have been devised solely by the author.